02/05
£4.99

BREAST
HEALTH

Dr. Miriam Stoppard

BREAST HEALTH

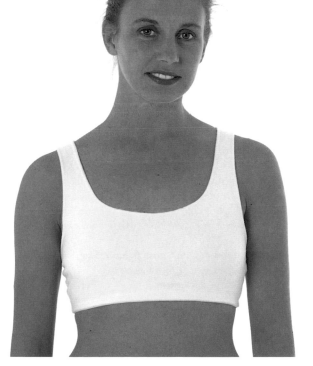

DORLING KINDERSLEY
London • New York • Sydney • Moscow

A DORLING KINDERSLEY BOOK

DESIGN & EDITORIAL   Mason Linklater

SENIOR MANAGING ART EDITOR   Lynne Brown
MANAGING EDITOR   Jemima Dunne

SENIOR ART EDITOR   Karen Ward
SENIOR EDITOR   Penny Warren

PRODUCTION   Antony Heller

First published in Great Britain in 1998

This revised edition published in Great Britain in 2003
by Dorling Kindersley Limited, 80 Strand
London WC2R 0RL

Visit us on the World Wide Web at http://www.dk.com

Material in this publication was previously published by
Dorling Kindersley in *The Breast Book*
by Dr. Miriam Stoppard.

A CIP catalogue record for this book is available
from the British Library.

ISBN 0-7513-6980-2

Reproduced in Singapore by Colourscan
Printed in Slovakia by Tlaciarne BB s.r.o.

CONTENTS

INTRODUCTION 6

INTRODUCTION

My overriding aim with this book is to help every woman to get to know her breasts, become unafraid of them and realize that their health is in her hands. Breasts are far from quiescent: throughout the whole of her fertile life, every woman experiences the monthly ebb and flow of their glandular tissues as clear evidence that her breasts are an integral part of her unique hormonal orchestra.

The female breast goes on maturing from puberty until the menopause, and its different elements mature in turn. Once you're aware of the normal phases of growth and shrinkage, you're liberated from fear and empowered to action. That's why it is so important for you to become familiar with your breasts.

Breast self-examination (BSE) is a simple way of getting to know how your breasts usually feel, so that you're alert to something unusual should it appear. Nine out of ten women don't do BSE, yet most who examine their breasts regularly will never find a lump, let alone a malignant one. I can only urge you to do BSE. It promotes breast awareness and makes you feel at home in your own body, so it's then easier to consult a doctor about anything untoward rather than just hoping it will go away.

Breast cancer takes up quite a large part of this book. Knowledge of risk and preventive factors can help you to reduce your own risk with life choices, such as having your first baby before 30, and lifestyle changes, such as keeping your weight down. No woman remains untouched by finding a new lump in her breast or having a suspicious shadow show up on a routine mammogram. I implore every woman to report breast symptoms early. Don't put it off. The chances are that whatever you've found is *not* cancer; but, most important, if it is, early diagnosis and treatment mean that the probability of a cure is high.

BREAST CARE

A woman's breasts undergo some of the most visible
and radical development of any part of her body. Indeed,
breasts continue to change even after they are fully grown.
A basic knowledge of the elements that make up your
breasts and their working parts will prepare you
to face a lifetime of changes with confidence.
The health of your breasts is in your hands, too.
It's important for your emotional well-being as well as
your physical health that you take on the responsibility of
caring for them, particularly by doing regular breast
self-examination (BSE) and, later, with regular
screening. This way, you'll be doing the best you can
to keep your breasts healthy all through your life.

ANATOMY OF THE BREAST

The breasts sit outside the ribcage and the pectoral muscles, and are cushioned by a layer of fat. This surrounds their working parts – the glandular tissue that contains the lobes and ducts.

The inner surface of the breasts lies closely against the pectoral muscles. The breasts extend vertically from the second to the sixth rib and horizontally from the breastbone across the ribcage, with an extension into the armpits. This extension is called the axillary tail.

The proportion of glandular tissue tends to be higher in young women. Older women have a higher proportion of fat in their breasts.

It's the fat that determines the size and shape of the breasts. The pectoral muscles, when well developed, also marginally influence breast size.

KNOW YOUR BREASTS

With a good understanding of the workings of the breast, a woman can learn to recognize when a problem needs medical attention. Then, if it does, she can get a feel for the treatment options that are open to her, participate fully in discussions with her doctor about the possibilities, and take an active role in deciding on the ultimate line of therapy for any conditions that may arise.

ELEMENTS OF THE BREAST

Breasts have two main components: the glandular elements, comprising the lobes and ducts, and the connective tissue that forms the supporting structure. Both of these elements are literally floating in fat, which at body temperature is liquid and accounts for most of breast volume.

The breast merges imperceptibly with the body fat around it, except for the part that extends into the armpit, the axillary tail, which pierces the upper layers of the muscles of the chest wall.

Lobes and ducts Each breast is divided into lobes of glandular tissue, where milk is produced, and each of these lobes contains 15–25 milk or lactiferous ducts, which lead towards the nipple. Some of them join together on the way, and each duct widens to form a collecting sac (lactiferous ampulla) just behind the nipple.

The nipple and areola While the skin covering the breast is smoother, thinner and more translucent than on most of the rest of the body, the skin of the areola is thinner still and contains complex sweat and sebaceous glands (these secrete an oily lubricating substance called sebum) and hair follicles. The surface of the areola is marked by a number of small bumps, called the tubercles of Montgomery. These bumps are sweat and sebaceous glands. They become more prominent in the second half of the menstrual cycle and grow throughout pregnancy.

The nipple can be flat, round, conical or cylindrical in shape. Its colour comes from the pigmentation and thinness of its skin, and it is either soft or firm according to the tone of the smooth muscle fibres within it. These tiny muscles are quite complex: they are embedded in connective tissue and the fibres run in three different directions – around, across and up – and extend into the connective tissue of the areola. It is these muscle fibres that make the nipple so responsive to cold or sexual arousal and cause it to stand out during breastfeeding so that the baby can take it in his mouth; all the fibres contract at once and the nipple becomes firm, ridged and elongated while the areolar skin puckers markedly. The core of the nipple is pierced by 15–25 milk (or lactiferous) ducts and sinuses that open up at its tip. The nipple itself has many sebaceous glands that keep it lubricated during breastfeeding.

Blood supply The same major arteries that supply the chest wall also supply the breast. The axillary artery comes from the armpit (axilla) and supplies the outer half of the breast; the internal mammary artery passes from the neck down the chest and supplies the inner half of the breast. It is the drainage of blood from the breasts through a network of veins that is more significant, however. Malignant tumours of the breast can spread to the rest of the body by shedding cancer cells into the blood like leaves from a tree; wherever these cells settle, a secondary breast cancer can form. The veins from the breast take blood back to the heart via those of the armpit and rib spaces, and then into veins deeper within the chest.

Nerve supply The large number of sensory nerve-endings that carry signals such as touch, pain and temperature are responsible for the exquisite sensitivity of the areola, particularly the nipple. As well as sensory nerves, the breast enjoys the bonus of extra nerves from the autonomic nervous system, which controls involuntary body functions such as digestion and sweating. Autonomic nerves form the connection whereby stimulation of the nipple can cause arousal and erection of the clitoris. This phenomenon is reported by very many women – indeed, some women can achieve orgasm simply by stimulation of the nipple.

The breast's lymphatic drainage Within the breast there is a network of delicate lymphatic vessels (see p. 10). These vessels communicate with a network in the skin, especially around the nipple under the areola, and there may even be another deep sub-mammary collection of tiny lymph vessels that lie on the surface of the chest muscles.

The lymphatic channels within the breast eventually end in the lymph nodes in the armpit, called the axillary lymph nodes. These nodes receive and filter 75 percent of all the lymph from the breast. Of the rest, about 20 percent passes to the lymph nodes around the breastbone and the other five percent pass deeper into the chest (continued p. 10).

LYMPH DRAINAGE OF THE BREAST

Lymphatic fluid flows around the body, bathing cells and organs in the same way as oil lubricates an engine. It drains into regional collecting points – the lymph nodes – which filter it and attack harmful organisms, preventing most infection from passing into the bloodstream. Seventy-five percent of the lymphatics in the breast drain into the lymph nodes in the armpit and from there to those above the collarbone. Lymph nodes around the breastbone receive almost all the rest.

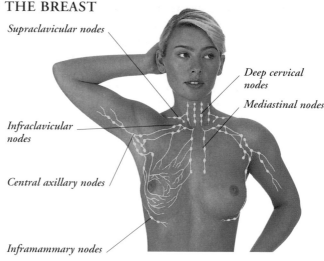

Supraclavicular nodes

Deep cervical nodes

Mediastinal nodes

Infraclavicular nodes

Central axillary nodes

Inframammary nodes

The lymphatic drainage of the breast is of particular importance because of its relevance to the diagnosis and treatment of breast cancer; the axillary lymph nodes can be affected if a cancer spreads through the lymphatic vessels from a primary tumour in the breast. This is why feeling for lumps in the armpit forms an essential part of breast self-examination (see pp. 14–17); you are not checking for tumours in these areas, but for swollen lymph nodes.

BREAST DEVELOPMENT

Although breast growth can't be seen until puberty, breast development begins very early in the embryo and can be discerned within just a few weeks of conception.

Adolescence The first external signs of breast development appear at the age of 10 or 11, although it can be as late as 14. The ovaries start to secrete oestrogen, leading to an accumulation of fat in the connective tissue that causes the breasts to enlarge. The duct system also begins to develop, but only to the point of forming cellular knobs at the end of the ducts. As far as doctors know, the mechanism that secretes milk doesn't develop until pregnancy.

The breasts may appear fully grown within a few years of puberty, but their development is not properly complete until their biological function is fulfilled – that is, until a woman carries a pregnancy to term and breastfeeds her baby, when the breasts will undergo further changes.

The ageing breast As women get older, the breasts tend to sag and flatten; the larger the breasts, the more they sag. With the menopause there is a reduction in stimulation by the hormone oestrogen to all tissues of the body, including breast tissue; this results in a reduction in the glandular tissue of the breasts so that they lose their earlier fullness. In some women, however, the menopause can bring with it an enormous increase in the size of the breasts.

Development and benign breast change As the various components of the breast continue to develop over the years, changes take place in all the tissues, which can give rise to lumps, cysts and sometimes nipple discharge. At one time these changes were thought of as diseases. Doctors no longer see them even as abnormal but simply as aberrations (or variations) of normal that are benign and require no treatment (see p. 26).

WHAT IS NORMAL?

All breasts are normal, regardless of size and shape. Other variations (usually due to quirks of development) are still common enough to be regarded as normal and harmless.

Hairs on the nipple There's hardly a woman who doesn't have at least one hair on her breasts, usually around the areola, and some women have many. Occasional shaving or plucking or using a depilatory cream is enough to remove them. Another option is permanent removal by electrolysis.

Inverted nipples In its usual form, the nipple is everted (turning outwards). Inverted nipples (turning inwards) are quite common, however, and are simply a variation of the norm, although they can be a cause of great concern for women. "Suction" devices such as nipple shells are widely available. A common worry is that breastfeeding will not be possible, but in fact the use of a breast shell can often solve this problem. It is possible to have cosmetic surgery to correct an inverted nipple. A previously everted nipple may become inverted as the result of nipple disease (see p. 36).

Asymmetry It is extremely rare for a woman's breasts to be entirely symmetrical; one is usually larger and consequently may be heavier and sit lower than the other. The difference between the right and left breast is rarely very great, but occasionally it is quite obvious. For some women, having asymmetrical breasts is of no concern but for others it is disconcerting and, if desired, can be corrected with plastic surgery, by enlarging one breast or by reducing the other.

LARGE BREASTS

How the breasts develop at puberty (see far left) depends on the sensitivity of breast tissue to the secretion of the hormone, oestrogen, which can vary among women.

Sometimes breast tissue can be hypersensitive to small amounts of oestrogen and the breasts enlarge and become heavy very rapidly, even making stretch marks in the skin.

The uncontrolled overgrowth of the breasts in pubescent girls is called juvenile or virginal hypertrophy. If unsupported, the suspensory ligaments that hold the breasts will become overstretched and the breasts will sag. Very heavy breasts can become pendulous even with good support.

Teenage girls who have extremely large breasts should be informed of the possibility of surgical breast reduction and offered counselling. The results of the operation are usually very good.

Moving the nipple and areolar skin is a part of such operations and it may affect the ability to breastfeed, although this depends on the surgical technique used. Ask your surgeon about operations that can preserve the milk ducts.

SUN PROTECTION

The breasts of white-skinned women can very easily become sunburned because the chest skin contains few melanocytes. These are the cells that protect the skin from sunburn by producing the tanning pigment, melanin.

• *Until a tan has become well established, you should apply a sun block with a sun protection factor (SPF) greater than 15 every two hours or so and after swimming or being in water.*

• *A gentle run-in period will help the skin accommodate itself to the bright ultraviolet rays. Have no more than five minutes' exposure on the first day, no more than ten minutes on the second, and a further five minutes on each day after that, up to half an hour.*

• *Even after this regime, you may be sunburned if you expose your breasts to sun for longer than two hours before they are given the opportunity to tan slowly.*

EVERYDAY BREAST CARE

The breasts don't need much in the way of beauty routines, but they do need to be treated with care, since their skin is extremely delicate. While many "beauty" treatments for the breasts exist, these are generally entirely worthless.

SKIN CARE

The skin of the breasts, particularly over the areola and the nipple (see p. 8), is thinner and more translucent than elsewhere on the body because the lower layers contain less collagen. This delicate skin needs to be treated gently, and should never be subjected to scrubbing or rough towelling since this can make the nipples sore and tender, particularly in the week prior to menstruation. The nipple and areola may become dry and flake premenstrually, so it's a good idea to moisturize them twice a week by gently massaging in an unperfumed moisturizer. If you are white-skinned and want to expose your breasts to the sun, make sure they are properly protected (see left).

Eczema can occur on the nipples. If you get a persistent patch, consult your doctor for a precise diagnosis and specific treatment, since in rare cases it can be a symptom of a more serious condition – a form of very slow-growing cancer called Paget's disease (see column, p. 38).

CAN BEAUTY REGIMES HELP THE BREASTS?

When I was a girl, the favourite technique among my friends for keeping your breasts pert was to bathe them first with hot water and then with cold water. This puckered up the areola and made the nipple erect, which was perhaps taken as a sign of uplift. It represented only a change in the slackness of the skin, however, and a transient one at that.

All kinds of beauty products are peddled in the hope of convincing women that potions, lotions and creams rubbed into the skin will help them keep the shape of their breasts or even increase their size. In fact, the only way to maintain the shape of the breasts is to start wearing a bra as soon as there's any weight in them. Nothing applied to the skin can alter their shape or consistency, both of which are determined by your own individual response to oestrogens secreted during puberty and thereafter with each menstrual cycle. Your breasts can be changed only from the inside, by the hormones manufactured inside your body.

BREAST EXERCISES

Exercises won't actually change the shape or size of your breasts. What you can achieve with exercise is to strengthen and tone your pectoral muscle. The suspensory ligaments supporting the breasts are attached to the pectoral muscle, so it's just about conceivable that exercises to tone this muscle could lift the breasts maybe 1 centimetre (½ inch) or thicken the pad of muscle on which the breasts sit, thereby increasing your bust measurement by perhaps 2 centimetres (¾ inch). If you're interested in increments of this order, try these exercises. You will need to do them regularly.

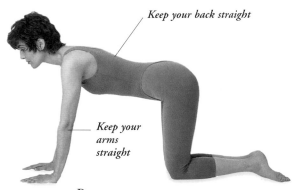

Keep your back straight

Keep your arms straight

PUSH-UPS

1 Kneel comfortably on all fours, with your hands shoulder-width apart and your palms flat on the floor.

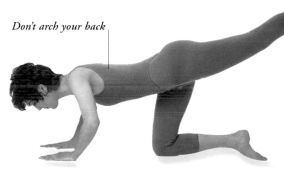

Don't arch your back

Keep your leg straight

2 Stretch your left leg out behind you with your toes pointing back. Bend your elbows to lower your chest nearly to the floor, keeping your shoulders in line with your hands. Repeat this several times, then repeat the whole sequence with your right leg out behind.

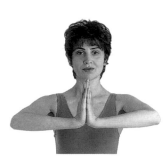

Palm presses
Press the palms and heels of your hands together in front of your breasts. Hold for five seconds. Repeat ten times.

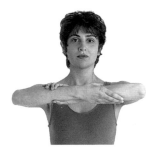

Forearm grip
Grasp your forearms with your hands at shoulder level and pull outwards without letting go. Repeat ten times.

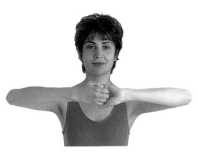

Finger lock
Curl your fingers, lock them together at shoulder level and pull outwards. Hold for five seconds. Repeat ten times.

ABOUT BREAST SELF-EXAMINATION (BSE)

Most women who regularly examine their breasts will never find a lump, let alone a malignant (harmful) one. Breast self-examination (BSE) is simply a way to explore your body and become familiar with it. You don't have to feel that you're looking for anything in particular; you're simply getting to know what your breasts usually feel and look like so that you can recognize something unusual if it appears. Every girl should start doing BSE as soon as she develops breasts and keep on doing it until she dies. There should be no time when you stop or interrupt this routine.

WOMEN WHO DO

Research shows that women who do breast self-examination have a positive attitude to life and to BSE; they think it's a good thing to do, and they're right. They are likely to be better educated, younger and in higher socio-economic groups than women who don't examine their breasts. They also engage in other preventive health measures such as having regular cervical smears and dental checkups.

Women who do BSE feel that breast cancer is the worst imaginable disease to affect women, but they're optimistic about the likelihood of being cured with early treatment and believe it is something they can control by doing BSE regularly. They don't think that doing BSE will inevitably lead to finding a cancerous lump and so they don't feel nervous about doing it. This is the kind of approach and attitude you should try to cultivate.

WOMEN WHO DON'T

Unfortunately, nine out of ten women don't do BSE. There are many reasons for this. Good information on BSE is hard to find and poor information tends to make women anxious. Even many health professionals who can tell you how to examine your breasts are unclear about what you're looking for because they're uncertain themselves. Not every health educator is a good communicator, and you may end up with a confusing message. Many books and pamphlets tell you that you have to look for a change but don't explain what the precise changes are. You have no clear idea, therefore, of what you're searching for, and that in itself provokes

"I love examining my breasts. I'm proud of them, and I want them to be healthy. It makes me feel I'm in control of my life."

Sue, 25, Musician

anxiety. Normal findings, such as premenstrual lumpiness (see right), can be very frightening if you don't know that they are normal, and can put you off BSE, since whatever is causing the lumps seems to be widespread.

It seems rather surprising in this day and age that women can actually be embarrassed about touching their breasts, yet many women in their fifties and sixties – the age group for which breast cancer is most common – grew up with the view that it was somehow bad, except in the bath, for a woman to touch her own body. A woman who considers that it is somehow improper to touch, let alone examine, her breasts can remain unaware for a long time of dramatic changes, even large, ulcerating tumours.

Sometimes women are put off BSE because they feel that there can't be a positive outcome if they find something needing medical attention. Only very few of the lumps that cause concern turn out to be cancerous. And even when they do, most women with breast cancer don't die from it. Early detection of breast cancer vastly improves the chances of a cure. I feel there's great room for optimism because while you're doing BSE you're in control of your health.

WHEN TO DO BSE

Most authorities advocating BSE suggest that you perform your examination at the same time every month – ideally in the week after your menstrual period – so that you have a consistent basis for comparison. When you're starting, however, I'm in favour of your examining your breasts at different times of the month because they will change in consistency and texture as you go through your monthly menstrual cycle (see right). I feel that all women should be aware of these changes and know how their breasts feel to touch. I also believe that it is better to perform BSE more often – say every two weeks instead of once a month – in a low-key, relaxed way so that it quickly becomes a habit and part of your normal life.

You should never feel tyrannized by BSE; if you don't want to do it, or if you sometimes miss a month or two, no harm will befall you. If you find that the idea of examining your breasts yourself makes you anxious, go along regularly to your doctor, say every three months, so that he or she can perform the examination for you, and if appropriate take advantage of other early detection techniques such as mammograms (see pp. 20–21).

NORMAL LUMPINESS

Most women find that their breasts acquire what can only be described as lumpiness in the second half of the menstrual cycle, and this becomes easier to feel just prior to menstruation.

• *Normal lumpiness can be felt throughout the breast tissue rather than concentrated in one spot. The lumps are very tiny and separate – about the size, shape and texture of an orange pip – and they may be tender if squeezed. This is because they are swollen milk glands, ready to develop into lactating glands should you become pregnant.*

• *If you examine your breasts again during the week after menstruation, you will find that these tiny lumps simply fade away as the glands shrink. When you've got used to these cyclical changes in your breasts, there's no need to examine them often; once a fortnight or once a month will do.*

HOW TO DO BSE

There are two elements to breast self-examination: looking and feeling (palpation). You will need a warm place where you can have some privacy and be free from interruptions. Just before going to bed is a good time, or when you are about to have a bath or shower.

LOOKING AT THE BREASTS

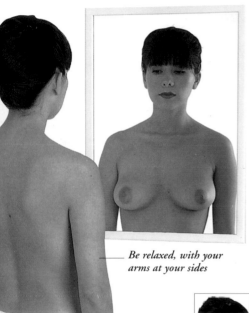

Don't forget to look at the upper part of the breast that leads into the armpit

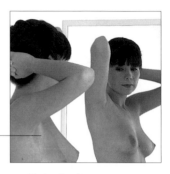

Be relaxed, with your arms at your sides

2 Raise both your arms above your head. Turn to one side so you can see your breasts in profile, and repeat your observations, as in Step 1. Do the same for the other side.

1 Undress to the waist and stand or sit in front of a mirror. Look at each breast carefully for changes in their appearance, size or the colour of the nipples; a difference in level between the nipples; patches of eczema on the nipples; or any dimpling of the skin.

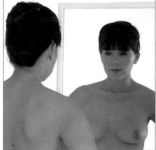

3 Turn to face the mirror. Place your hands firmly on your hips and press in hard. You should feel your chest muscles tense. Repeat your observations.

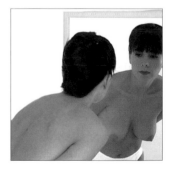

4 Now lean forward from the waist. Look again for dimpling or puckering of the skin, a change in outline of the breast or if the nipple appears to be drawn in.

FEELING THE BREASTS

1 Lie back in a relaxed position and put your right arm behind your head. This shifts the breast tissue towards the centre of your chest, giving you better access to it and making it easier to feel. If your breasts are very large, a pillow under your left shoulder may help.

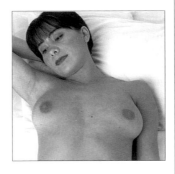

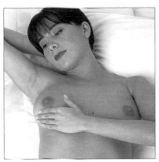

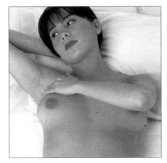

2 Touching firmly, use your left hand to examine your right breast. Use one of the patterns (right) or your own, as long as it's systematic.

3 Check your armpit and along the top of your collarbone for lumps (if the lymph nodes are swollen, you will feel them as lumps).

4 Put your left arm behind your head and, using your right hand, examine your left breast in the same systematic way. Remember to check the armpit and collarbone.

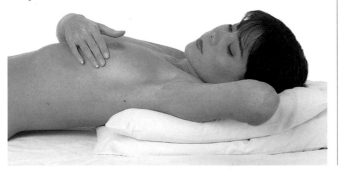

PATTERNS OF FEELING

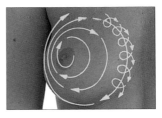

Concentric circles
Start with a big circle around the outside of the breast, making smaller circles with your fingers as you go around the breast. Work inwards until you reach the nipple.

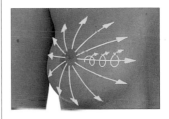

Radial pattern
Mentally divide the breast into a clock. Work out from the nipple towards 12 o'clock, then 1, 2, 3 o'clock and so on to check the whole breast.

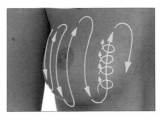

Up and down
Imagine the breast as a series of vertical bands; go up and down each one. Move your fingers in small circles as you work around the breast.

WHAT YOU MIGHT FIND

Above all, you are looking for a change in your breasts. You won't be able to recognize change, however, until you've examined your breasts a few times and established what is normal for you. Here are some of the things you may find in your breasts. They are all quite normal and healthy.

Lumps and pseudo-lumps   You may observe many subtle changes in your breasts. Cancer is not subtle, so don't panic over a very tiny and discrete lump, particularly if its size varies over your monthly cycle. Remember, your breasts may be lumpy naturally or pre-menstrually (see p. 15).

Losing weight often makes natural breast lumpiness more evident. The breastbone (between your breasts) makes joints at either edge with the ribs, which may be prominent. If you're very thin, one of the hard lumps that you feel could simply be breast tissue felt over the end of a rib.

You may feel a swelling of breast tissue between the nipple and the armpit, or directly above the nipple. During the pre-menstrual period, both of these areas are more likely to swell up and become tender. There is also a ridge of tissue in the lower part of the breast that feels thicker and more lumpy than other parts of the breast. Under the nipple is a hollow spot where the milk ducts rise to the surface.

Scar tissue from an infection or surgery (even a biopsy) will always remain as a palpable lump or ridge. (If your doctor examines your breasts, do mention this and the date it occurred, to avoid concern and unnecessary tests.)

Pain   Soreness and discomfort are extremely common in women's breasts (see p. 26). In the vast majority of cases they are connected with menstrual hormones, and they are very rarely symptoms of cancer. If soreness persists or if it is causing you problems, however, your doctor will be able to help, normally by prescribing oil of evening primrose.

Normal findings

When examining your breasts, you may find changes that cause you concern. Many of these things, however, are quite normal and healthy and are shown below. If you are at all worried about any changes, consult your doctor at once.

SIGNIFICANT CHANGES

Once you have been doing BSE long enough to get used to what is normal in your breasts, you will need to be on the alert for any changes that require a doctor's attention (there are several characteristic ones that might be of concern). First, when looking at your breasts, you might observe:

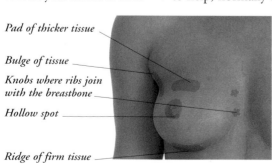

Pad of thicker tissue

Bulge of tissue

Knobs where ribs join with the breastbone

Hollow spot

Ridge of firm tissue

- veins that are visible through the skin more prominently than usual
- change in the size of either breast
- change in the colour or texture of the skin
- new dimpling or puckering of the skin over the breast and nipple, or change in the breast outline
- change in the appearance of the nipple such as redness, scaling, crusting or drawing in
- discharge or bleeding from the nipple.

When feeling, you are really looking for only one thing: a new, discrete lump that is constant in size and doesn't vary with your menstrual cycle. It may be attached to the skin, causing puckering, or fixed to the tissues deeper in the breast. If you feel such a lump, your next step should be to examine the armpit to see whether or not any of your lymph nodes are swollen, and run your finger along the top of your collarbone to see if there are any swollen nodes there too. There are three main criteria for deciding that a lump needs medical investigation:

- the lump is new
- it is very distinct, not just a thickening of breast tissue
- it is unchanged through one or two menstrual cycles.

If you find something but can't decide whether it's serious or not, see your doctor anyway, if only to set your mind at rest. The vast majority of lumps detected by BSE are not cancerous and are quite normal.

WHAT TO DO IF YOU FIND A LUMP

First, check the same part of the other breast. If what you have found is symmetrical, it's just the way your breasts are made and nothing for you to worry about. If the lump is asymmetrical, don't panic. Phone your doctor's surgery to make an appointment for a breast examination at the earliest opportunity. If he or she is at all worried, you will be referred very quickly to see a hospital specialist and further tests will be done (see p. 56). Make a mental note of exactly where the lump is in your breast and try not to keep feeling it to see if it's still there or if it's tender.

Now sit down, phone your best friend and ask her to come round straight away. However rational you think you can be about it, you will be glad of moral support before, during and after your medical appointment. Just keep on reminding yourself that the majority of breast lumps are not cancerous and turn out to be harmless.

DISCHARGE

Some pamphlets and books about BSE tell you to squeeze your nipples and check for discharge. You should not do this as part of your breast self-examination routine.

Squeezing the nipple can create discharge where there was none before, because it increases the hormone, prolactin, in the body, which in turn causes the breasts to produce liquid (although not proper milk).

The way to check for discharge is simply to examine your clothes, and you should do this at least every time you do BSE. Discharge is cause for concern only if it appears without any squeezing of the nipples, if it is persistent or if it's from one nipple only (gently squeeze your other nipple to check this). In all these cases, you should consult your doctor (see p. 36).

MAMMOGRAPHIC SCREENING

To have a mammogram done, you'll be asked to strip to the waist and remove any deodorant or talc from your breasts. The reason for this is that they may show up as microcalcifications (see p. 21).

You will then be asked to stand in front of the machine and the radiologist will compress your breast between two plates. The procedure is described as painless, but it is not without a degree of discomfort, particularly if the plates are cold; the sensation lasts no more than 10 or 15 seconds, however, so it's easily bearable. Two views of each breast will usually be taken.

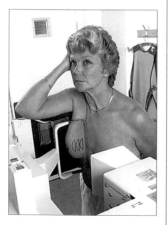

Obtaining the image
The radiologist compresses each breast in turn between two plates so that a good image is obtained.

SCREENING

Breast self-examination is recommended for all women, at all stages of their lives, but additional checks are advisable for older women, who have a higher risk of breast cancer, and for women in other high-risk groups – with breast cancer in the family, for instance. In the UK, there is a screening programme to make sure that women between 50 and 65 years of age attend screening clinics regularly. Screening involves having a physical breast examination – a doctor will examine your breasts in the same way that you do at home for BSE (see pp. 16–17) – and a mammogram (see left and below), which can detect smaller abnormalities of the breasts than a physical examination.

There now exists clear evidence that early detection by screening and treatment cuts down the number of women dying from breast cancer. Studies performed in Sweden and the USA have shown that screening can reduce by up to one-third deaths from breast cancer in women between the ages of 50 and 65. Early detection automatically means earlier treatment and therefore increases the chances of a full recovery if a lump is found that turns out to be breast cancer. Early detection also means that you can have greater choice in how your cancer will be treated.

It's understandable to feel anxious about having regular mammograms. However, it is likely that you will be one of the 99 women out of every 100 routinely screened who are found not to have cancer.

MAMMOGRAPHY

A mammogram is a low-dose X-ray of the breast. It is such a refined method of imaging the breast that it can pick up small cancers and other abnormalities that neither you nor your doctor can feel on manual examination.

Mammograms are not done with the same frequency in all age groups. Because breast cancer is comparatively rare in women under the age of 50, it is only after 50 that mammograms are recommended for screening purposes. Women who fall into high-risk groups will be offered annual mammograms at an earlier age than usual (see above). At present in the UK, mammography is offered to women over 50 years of age every three years, although there is currently some debate about whether it should be offered more frequently.

Mammography is less effective in women under 50, since their breast tissue is more dense and abnormalities don't show up so well, but it is still more sensitive than BSE. This is why it can be used as a diagnostic tool, to investigate a lump found in physical examination, for example, or to look for further lumps when one has already been found.

GETTING THE RESULTS

The films are developed and examined by a radiologist who specializes in interpreting mammograms. The results usually take only a few days to come through and most women will be told that they're fine and just need regular screening. A small number will be asked to come back for further tests. This can be worrying, but the chances of getting the all-clear are still high. Although mammograms are good for detecting small lumps, they're not much use in determining a lump's precise character, so extra tests may be needed.

Microcalcifications These are tiny deposits of calcium that show up as very fine specks on a mammogram. They may be quite normal and many women have them but, because they have been linked with cancer in a small number of cases, the radiologist will always mention their presence. They are only worrying if they suddenly appear in a cluster in one breast. If it's your first mammogram, your doctor may wait a year before doing another one to see if there's any change. If the pattern of microcalcification appears very abnormal, a biopsy will be carried out at once (see p. 56).

Lumps If your mammogram shows any kind of lump, further tests will be necessary. A lump that's large enough to feel easily with your fingers can be aspirated by inserting a fine needle to draw off some of the tissue. This is called fine-needle aspiration cytology, or FNAC (see p. 33).

If the lump is fluid-filled, it's a cyst (see p. 35), which is nearly always perfectly harmless; your specialist will draw off the fluid with a needle and will usually discard it. If it's solid, some of the cells that have been drawn off will be smeared on a slide, stained, and examined in the laboratory.

If the lump isn't easy to feel, you will probably have an ultrasound scan (see p. 22) to determine whether it's a solid lump or a cyst. Either way it will be investigated with FNAC or core needle biopsy (see p. 56). When a lump can't be felt, both of these specimens are taken with the guidance of ultrasound so that the tumour can be precisely located.

"After my first screening session, I felt ambivalent really. You know, glad that nothing was found but scared that something will show up next time."

Claire, 53,
Tour Operator

OTHER IMAGING TECHNIQUES

Mammography is the most widely used method of imaging the breast, but there are some other techniques that you may come across, particularly if you are referred for other tests after a routine screening mammogram.

XERO-MAMMOGRAPHY

Xero-mammography requires different equipment from the standard X-ray machine that takes a mammogram. It is not necessarily any more accurate than mammography; it just gives a different end-product: an image on paper rather than on film. Accuracy of interpretation depends on the experience of the radiologist, whatever method is used.

ULTRASOUND

Many of us have come across the painless ultrasonic scans during pregnancy. Ultrasound can produce a picture very similar to an X-ray photograph. The patterns are produced by the echoes of sound waves, which vary in intensity according to the solidity of the tissue that they bounce off. Ultrasound can be particularly useful when examining very dense breasts, so it's good for younger women, and it can detect very small lumps that can't yet be felt, particularly tiny cysts. It's very accurate with larger, palpable lumps, and it can distinguish between solid lumps and those that are filled with fluid. Ultrasound also detects calcification (see p. 21), and can show up the blood supply to a tumour; a rich supply of blood is characteristic of cancerous lumps.

THERMOGRAPHY

Less familiar than X-rays or ultrasound, this is never a first-line investigation. The heat-sensitive photographs usually support manual examination and mammography.

Rapidly growing and dividing tissue such as cancer has a higher temperature than the tissue that surrounds it. Thermography works by mapping out the temperatures in different tissues, so a growing cyst or a tumour will show up on a thermogram as a more intense area of heat than its surroundings. The patient undresses and holds her arms up or stretched out from her body to allow the breast skin to cool. Photographs are then taken with an infrared camera.

BENIGN BREAST CHANGES

Many changes in the breast reflect quite normal,
harmless conditions. Such changes do not
necessarily indicate cancer or even disease.
A woman should be helped to maintain a calm and
rational response to benign breast changes, such as cyclical
and non-cyclical pain, cysts, solid lumps and nipple
discharge, and be reassured as to diagnosis and options for
treatment, if it is needed. For her own peace of mind and
well-being, a woman needs to understand that benign
breast changes are simply the normal effects of
her age, menstrual cycle and lifestyle.

CHANGE OR DISEASE?

Cysts, solid lumps and nipple discharge are all normal, harmless conditions that arise in the breast. Since there's no abnormality present, it's misleading to call such conditions "diseases", and well-informed doctors now use the term "benign breast change". This is crucial to a woman for whom the word disease implies something abnormal or dangerous. It's imperative that doctors too stop thinking of these conditions as disease because they have been trained to believe that disease justifies intervention. If your doctor refers to a breast condition in ambiguous terms, always ask for clarification of the terminology. Defer treatment until you have a second opinion if you don't understand.

A NEW APPROACH TO CLASSIFICATION

Until about 18 years ago, breast conditions were not well understood and there was confusion as to what was normal and what was abnormal. In 1980, researchers in Cardiff, Wales, developed a new and logical classification system for breast conditions that has a scientific basis. This system relates the most common breast conditions to normal changes that take place in the breast throughout a woman's lifetime, and has been accepted in most countries where breast research takes place, including the US and the UK. It provides a rational explanation for practically all benign breast conditions. The Cardiff researchers decided to rename benign breast conditions as Aberrations (changes) of Normal Development and Involution (shrinkage), giving the acronym ANDI.

WHY ANDI?

The ANDI classification is based on two facts about benign breast conditions. First, most conditions relate to the normal pattern of breast development with its stages of growth and shrinkage. Second, each condition fits into one of the three main periods of women's fertile lives (puberty to 25 years, 25 to 35 years and 35 to 55 years), so certain symptoms are more common at certain ages.

Take the development of a fibroadenoma (see p. 34) for example. Common in teenagers and women in their 20s, this lump is nothing more than a breast lobule of unusual size, shape and consistency. Under a microscope, the cells from a normal lobule and a fibroadenoma look identical.

Your age is therefore of particular importance if you discover a breast lump. Under the age of 35, the chances are overwhelmingly that you've found a fibroadenoma, which is benign and nothing to worry about. If you're between the ages of 35 and 55, the chances are that the lump is an innocent cyst. But if you're over the age of 55, cancer must be a possibility and your doctor will take immediate steps to make a firm diagnosis.

In the light of these observations, doctors can now interpret the majority of benign breast conditions as age-related variations on the normal; they are therefore better thought of as aberrations or "mistakes" rather than diseases. Such aberrations for most women are symptomless, so they rarely prompt you to consult a doctor. Only a few cause symptoms such as pain (see right), and even fewer lead to disease. Most never get beyond the state of being simply a variation on normal development.

ANDI AND DISEASE

There is no evidence that aberrations inevitably progress to disease. On the contrary, it seems that for this to happen some additional factor is needed – often an external one, such as smoking or an excessive alcohol intake. Duct ectasia (see p. 36), for instance, rarely if ever goes on to infection or an abscess except where a woman smokes.

ANDI, therefore, usefully defines the spectrum from normal to minor aberrations that encompasses most benign breast conditions. Disease, on the other hand, is associated with other possibly external triggers (see pp. 43–48).

YOUR CONCERNS

Almost all women fear breast cancer, so any breast symptom can cause alarm. Indeed, most women with breast symptoms seek reassurance even before they consider treatment. The women most at risk, and therefore those who should be most concerned about breast cancer, are those who are under 50 years old with a first-degree relative (that is, mother or sister) who developed breast cancer at a young age. If you know you have a high risk of developing breast cancer or are especially worried about your breasts, ask your family doctor for referral to a special breast clinic; it's your right to do so. Should you develop breast cancer, don't accept treatment from a general surgeon who treats fewer than 30 breast cancers a year.

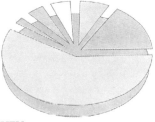

KEY

▷	65%	LUMP, WITH OR WITHOUT PAIN
▷	16%	PAIN (MASTALGIA)
▷	8%	PAINFUL LUMPINESS
▷	5%	NIPPLE DISCHARGE
▷	4%	OTHER
▷	2%	NIPPLE RETRACTION

Breast symptoms
The vast majority of benign breast disorders give rise to three main symptoms: a lump or lumpiness, pain and nipple discharge. Taken singly, breast pain is the most common complaint women report: at one breast clinic it appeared in 170 out of 480 women (35 percent). But not all women who suffer breast pain ever seek help for it; it's thought that seven out of ten women suffer to some degree from breast pain, tenderness and lumpiness.

SEE A BREAST SPECIALIST IF...

Pain is not the only symptom that should make you visit a breast specialist. Any of these symptoms will require further investigation and you should not be put off seeking the necessary help and advice. See a breast specialist if:

● *your pain is associated with a breast lump; pain doesn't respond to your doctor's treatment; you are post-menopausal and have persistent pain in one breast.*

● *you find a new, discrete lump or a new lump in pre-existing general lumpiness; a cyst persistently refills after being drained; you notice asymmetrical lumpiness at the beginning of your menstrual cycle for more than one cycle.*

● *you have nipple discharge associated with a lump; there is sufficient discharge to stain your clothes; you have bloodstained, persistent or painful discharge.*

BREAST PAIN

Is breast pain real? To the 60 percent of women who experience mastalgia, to give breast pain its medical name, the question seems ludicrous. Of course it's real – so real that for some women just having the breasts touched can be excruciating. Less than 20 years ago, however, breast pain, like gynaecological pain such as menstrual cramps, was thought to be all in the mind; for decades it had been labelled neurotic, hysterical and psychosomatic.

The unsympathetic and largely masculine trend of labelling breast pain as "a nervous disorder" was started in the nineteenth century by an eminent British surgeon, Astley Cooper, but was still widespread in the 1950s and 1960s. It was not until 1978 that Professor Robert Mansel of Cardiff, Wales, investigated this notion and reported that mastalgia sufferers were indeed psychologically stable and deserved a sympathetic approach to treatment. Largely due to Mansel's work, breast pain has become recognized as a legitimate complaint.

Breast pain can be classified into two types: cyclical, which is associated with menstrual periods (see pp. 28–30), and non-cyclical. Non-cyclical pain may originate in the breast or in the nearby muscles and joints, in which case it is not true breast pain (see p. 30).

Treating women with breast pain Studies carried out in Manchester, England, indicate that women suffering from breast pain don't always get the understanding and treatment they deserve; and it's clear that too many women seeking help aren't being examined or treated appropriately. Although more than half the women studied had seen their family doctor, they still needed help and treatment. Other women avoided their doctor out of fear or embarrassment. Still others had been met with the attitude that breast pain was a "nervous" or "neurotic" disorder.

It is still common for doctors to prescribe ineffective remedies – diuretics or even antibiotics – to treat mastalgia. Some doctors suggest evening primrose oil, which is widely available in over-the-counter products, although evening primrose oil is effective only in high doses that are expensive unless obtained on prescription (see p. 29).

Effects on lifestyle Although mastalgia can significantly disrupt daily life and even be incapacitating, not all women feel justified in consulting a doctor about it. In one study,

60 percent of women said that they felt they had to cope without medical help. Although women may be reluctant to consult a doctor, the pain often causes them to ring a breast helpline – indeed, mastalgia is the most common reason for women calling such a helpline. Researchers in the UK have demonstrated just how seriously breast pain can interfere with normal daily life. The following figures give the percentages of women who suffered from varying degrees of breast pain:

• sufficient pain to make them particularly aware of the breasts: 42%
• discomfort wearing a bra or light clothing: 26%
• uncomfortable running up or down stairs: 19%
• too uncomfortable for close physical contact: 17%
• cannot bear any physical contact or pressure; pain would interrupt sleep and preclude sex: 9%.

Fear and breast pain Even if breast pain does not interfere radically with normal life, fear of breast pain can be crippling because sufferers fear that cancer is the cause. Studies from Cardiff demonstrate that almost nine out of ten women with mastalgia are much more worried about the possibility of cancer than about the pain itself. This includes the one in six women who suffers from incapacitating pain.

It's reasonable to be fearful of getting breast cancer, but it's not reasonable to be paranoid about it. If you have breast pain and are worried about it, you should visit your doctor. Bear in mind, though, that breast pain is rarely a symptom of breast cancer. And it would be very wrong indeed to think that the worse the pain, the greater the chance that it's caused by malignancy (a cancerous tumour). In fact, the opposite is true. The worse the pain, the less likely it is to be due to a malignant growth. Looked at this way, breast pain is a reassuring symptom since its presence all but excludes breast cancer.

Psychology and breast pain All breast conditions can give rise to anxiety. For many women the symptoms are stressful in their own right, and as such may lead to psychological disorders. On the other hand, psychological disorders may show up as – or be the cause of – breast symptoms, although in saying this I am not suggesting for a moment that the symptoms are imaginary.

Ironically, the highest levels of anxiety are found in women who are subsequently diagnosed as having purely benign disorders. Studies using internationally accepted

Locations of pain
Pain that seems to be in the breast may in fact originate from some other part of the body, typically the bones or muscles. Locating the pain precisely helps a doctor decide whether the pain is true breast pain.

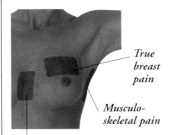

True breast pain

Musculo-skeletal pain

Musculoskeletal pain

DIAGNOSING CYCLICAL PAIN

One of the first things your doctor will want to establish is whether the pain is cyclical or not.

A chart known as the standard Cardiff chart allows you to record your pain each day – whether there is no pain, mild pain or severe pain – so that you and your doctor can see whether a pattern emerges.

The first day of each menstrual period is marked with a tick. Put a cross through any dates that don't apply (such as 29 February). After a couple of months, the relationship between the menstrual cycle and breast pain will emerge.

methods for measuring anxiety also came up with the startling finding that the degree of stress felt by women with severe mastalgia is similar to that felt by women with operable breast cancer on the morning of surgery.

Given this degree of pain and anxiety, it is very important for women to realize that they can receive simple and effective treatment for mastalgia.

Lumpiness and breast pain It used to be thought that breast lumpiness, including cyclical lumpiness (see p. 15), could cause breast pain and that, conversely, breast pain would eventually lead to lumpiness. Neither of these concepts has any medical foundation whatsoever. When mammography was used to measure lumpiness, it was found that women with severe lumpiness had no more breast pain than women with no lumpiness at all. Then again, when women with mastalgia had ultrasound examinations, only half had lumpy breasts. Nor does the degree of lumpiness reflect the degree of pain that a woman experiences. Both lumpiness and pain are common, however, so it is hardly surprising that they often occur together. The association between pain and lumpiness is mainly true of cyclical pain.

As well as lumpiness, breast pain is commonly associated with swelling, hardening and a feeling of tension in the breast. Your doctor may refer to this as engorgement, but it's not the same as the engorgement a breastfeeding mother experiences when her breasts become over-full with milk.

CYCLICAL BREAST PAIN

The commonest kind of breast pain is associated with the menstrual cycle and is nearly always related to fluctuations in hormone levels that every woman experiences as part of the cycle. Pain is probably related to the sensitivity of breast tissue to hormones and this can differ within a breast and between your two breasts. Hormones aren't the whole story, however, because in the majority of women the pain is more severe in one breast than in the other. Most women experience some degree of breast pain when their breasts become sensitive just prior to menstruation. Some women, however, may experience soreness and tenderness starting in the middle of the cycle with ovulation and continuing for about two weeks until menstruation takes place. Others find that this pre-menstrual soreness becomes even worse after the birth of their first child.

The degree of pain varies. Sometimes it's hardly noticeable, but for some women the pain is so great that they wince when hugged, can't stand to wear anything tight around their breasts and can't lie on their stomachs. Sometimes the pain spreads out towards the armpit and occasionally down the arm to the elbow, which can cause women to fear that the pain is due to cancer or heart disease.

Causes of cyclical pain There are many theories as to how hormones may be responsible for causing cyclical breast pain. One possibility is that the pain is due to changes in the production of prolactin, the milk-producing hormone, in response to changes in levels of thyroid hormone. We know that some women are very sensitive to thyroxine and respond to it by producing very high levels of prolactin, which induces breast pain. It's thought that abnormal "pulses" of prolactin may underlie cyclical mastalgia.

Breast pain can be affected by stress, and another theory suggests that it may be related to the many hormones that flood the body during stress. These include adrenaline, noradrenaline, hydrocortisone and thyroid hormone.

French research has shown that mastalgia may occur when there's a lowered production of progesterone, thus changing the normal ratio of progesterone to oestrogen in the second half of the menstrual cycle. Not all doctors agree with this theory, or with the practice of using progesterone to treat mastalgia. At the times in women's lives when hormonal swings are greatest (during puberty, pregnancy or the menopause) breast pain may be intense. During the menopause this may be caused by the ovaries secreting oestrogen without producing progesterone; this changes the normal ratio of progesterone to oestrogen.

Treating cyclical breast pain If a man suffered breast pain 13 times a year, he wouldn't hesitate to demand effective treatment. Neither should you. I believe that every woman with mastalgia has the right to try evening primrose oil, which is effective and safe, on prescription.

Evening primrose oil has to be taken in a large dose (three grams daily) to be effective. It also needs to be taken over a long period of time since its effect builds slowly – in most cases it takes as long as four months to see if there is a good response to the treatment. Notwithstanding the large dose and prolonged usage, evening primrose oil has very few side-effects, which is why it should be the first-line treatment of choice (continued p. 30).

SEQUENCE OF TREATMENTS

If your doctor establishes that your pain is not cyclical, it will be treated according to cause (see pp. 30–31). If it is cyclical, there are a number of possible treatments.

- *For mild pain, reassurance is often all that is required.*

- *For severe pain, your doctor will first prescribe evening primrose oil.*

- *If pain persists, your doctor may go on to danazol.*

- *If danazol is ineffective, bromocriptine may be tried.*

- *If there is no response and you still have severe pain, your doctor may try hormone treatment with tamoxifen or goserelin (see pp. 79 and 80).*

SELF-HELP FOR CYCLICAL PAIN

Although I firmly believe that all women with mastalgia should receive medical treatment if they want it, there are self-help remedies that are worth trying. The following remedies are in no way dangerous and are easy to implement.

• *Vitamin E is said to help, although this is unproven.*

• *Water retention doesn't cause cyclical mastalgia, but it can make it seem worse if you're generally retaining fluid pre-menstrually.*

• *If you're bothered by water retention, you might try taking naturally occurring diuretics such as parsley and capsicums (sweet peppers). Coffee is one of the most powerful natural diuretics known and could greatly help to eliminate fluid.*

• *Early research suggests that a diet low in animal fat can reduce cyclical mastalgia. Although this is still unproven, such a diet is healthy anyway.*

Danazol – a drug that blocks ovulation – has a success rate of nearly 80 percent and this makes it the ideal second-line treatment. Despite its success it is not suitable for everyone: some women may experience side-effects such as weight gain and irregular periods. Danazol is given in a dose of 200 milligrams daily for two months; if it has been effective after this time the dose will be gradually reduced.

Bromocriptine works by blocking the hormone prolactin, and may be advised for women who have not responded to evening primrose oil. It has about the same success rate as treatment with evening primrose oil, but it is more likely to have side-effects – nausea, vomiting and headache are among the most common. Giving it in a low dose at first (1.25 milligrams nightly) and gradually increasing the dose to 2.5 milligrams twice daily can help to avoid these. You should always take bromocriptine with food.

NON-CYCLICAL BREAST PAIN

There are two types of non-cyclical breast pain: true breast pain, which comes from the breast but is unrelated to the menstrual cycle, and pain that is felt in the region of the breast but is actually coming from somewhere else. This latter kind nearly always involves the muscles, bones or joints and for this reason it is called musculoskeletal pain (see Locations of pain, p. 27). Two-thirds of non-cyclical mastalgia is pain of musculoskeletal origin. Sometimes what appears to be breast pain is due to underlying lung or gallbladder disease.

Diagnosing non-cyclical pain Non-cyclical breast pain is relatively uncommon and feels quite unlike cyclical breast pain. It doesn't vary with your menstrual cycle at all and is entirely unrelated to hormones. It's nearly always confined to one spot and you can usually point to exactly where the pain is – it's impossible to do this with cyclical breast pain. Keeping a record of your pain on a daily pain chart (see column, p. 28) over a period of months will show that there is no cyclical pattern and that the pain is therefore unrelated to menstruation.

If your doctor suspects non-cyclical pain while examining you, you may be asked to lean forward so that the breast falls away from the chest. This helps to clarify whether the pain is located in the breast or in the chest wall. As with cyclical pain, a proper diagnosis is important otherwise you may worry needlessly about breast cancer or your heart.

True non-cyclical breast pain   There are some benign breast conditions that may be associated with true breast pain. Burning or stabbing pains centred around or under the nipple are nearly always caused by ectasia (see Dilatation of the milk ducts, p. 36) and tend to run an intermittent, although harmless, course.

A tender spot accompanied by occasional stabbing pain or an ache is common. Its cause is unknown, but it is no reason for anxiety. The pain can be relieved by an injection of local anaesthetic mixed with prednisone, which will help to reduce any inflammation. A cyst (see p. 35) occasionally underlies a tender spot.

Pain of non-breast origin   Pain originating in the chest wall or spine may be felt in the breast area. The most usual cause is a form of arthritis, called costochondritis, which affects the ends of the ribs where they join the breastbone; this condition is called Tietze's syndrome. If your pain is worse when you take a deep breath or press on your breastbone and ribs, it's likely to be this kind of arthritis. Taking an analgesic (painkiller) such as paracetamol or a non-steroidal anti-inflammatory drug like ibuprofen is often effective, so confirming the diagnosis.

Very occasionally pain felt close to the breast originates from a pinched nerve in the neck. An X-ray of the cervical spine will reveal a condition called spondylosis, the natural erosion of the joints between the vertebrae due to ageing. Another possibility is spondylitis, which means that there's some inflammation of the inter-vertebral joints.

In both of these conditions, spurs of new bone are laid down on the sides of the vertebrae and press on the nerves. The resulting pain may be felt in the neck, shoulder, chest, arm or hand. Treatment includes analgesics to relieve the pain, manipulation and physiotherapy, and exercises that are specifically designed to strengthen the muscles of the neck and shoulders.

Although rare, inflammation in the veins of the breast, called Mondor's syndrome, causes pain very like that of an infection or an abscess (you may also hear your doctor use the word phlebitis, which means inflammation of a vein). Careful examination may reveal the inflamed vein, which feels a bit like a string under your fingertips. This condition is not harmful – a blood clot hardly ever escapes from an inflamed vein. Treated with hot and cold compresses and analgesics, it will settle down in about a week.

SELF-HELP FOR ANY BREAST PAIN

For any breast pain, whether it's cyclical or non-cyclical in origin, the following ideas are well worth trying.

- *Invest in a good support bra that is comfortable enough to wear at night.*

- *Consider learning mental techniques such as deep relaxation, meditation and visualization. Some women find them helpful.*

- *Hypnosis is still controversial, but with an expert practitioner results can be as good as with oil of evening primrose.*

*If you consult your family
doctor with a breast lump,
you will be referred to a
breast specialist who will first
try to establish whether the
lump is benign or malignant.*

*To do this, doctors use a "triple
assessment" approach to check
out the lump: that is, manual
examination, mammography
or ultrasound, and fine-needle
aspiration cytology (see column,
right).*

*Physical examination alone
won't reveal whether the lump
is filled with fluid or solid. An
ultrasound scan will make this
distinction, however, and may
pick up other lumps that are
too small to feel.*

*If microscopic examination
reveals malignant cells, your
doctor will move on to a biopsy
(see p. 58). Surgeons will
remove any lump in the breast
of a post-menopausal woman
regardless of whether the cells
are benign or malignant.*

Physical examination
Your doctor will note the
location of the lump in one
of four quadrants (see below)
and examine your armpits for
swollen lymph nodes.

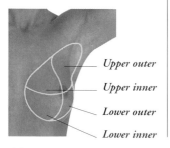

Upper outer

Upper inner

Lower outer

Lower inner

BREAST LUMPS

The commonest breast lumps belong to a group of
harmless conditions that have no sinister implications
whatsoever, but can cause anxiety if you don't understand
how they arise and develop. Every woman has a lump (or
general lumpiness) of one sort or another, although it may
often be too small to feel. Practically all lumps are merely a
variation of normal; they do not develop into cancers and
they won't kill you. There is no actual disease. This is very
important information for all women because on
discovering a lump in their breasts they can be reassured
that it probably belongs in the harmless category.

There are only two kinds of common benign breast
lump: fibroadenomas (see p. 34) and cysts (see p. 35).
These lumps are not diseases – they are part of the normal
changing growth pattern of the breasts throughout
women's lives (see p. 24). There is a third type of lump
called a pseudo-lump which, as its name implies, isn't really
a breast lump at all. A pseudo-lump can occur at any age
and is nearly always extreme normal lumpiness, but it
should be checked to make certain that all is well. (Other
pseudo-lumps, such as the end of a rib or scar tissue, are
discussed on page 18.)

Doctors have no idea why these non-cancerous lumps
appear, although they're probably related in some way to
natural fluctucations in hormone production. Cysts and
fibroadenomas grow only during a woman's fertile years,
although they may be detected years later. They occur at
opposite ends of the hormonal spectrum, fibroadenomas
being most common in the early part of a woman's fertile
life and cysts during mid-fertile life.

Lumpiness A special word needs to be said about lumpy
breasts. Lumpiness in both breasts is never sinister and
needs no treatment, especially if it's worse pre-menstrually.
Some doctors still dub it fibrocystic disease, which all
experts agree is an alarmist misnomer. The danger is that
some doctors still believe fibrocystic disease to be generally
precancerous, whereas this is very rarely so. Once a doctor
is thinking this way, however, preventive measures may be
recommended to you – even bilateral mastectomy
(complete removal of both breasts). If your doctor suggests
this, get a second opinion from a breast specialist. Bilateral
mastectomy is hardly ever justified for lumpy breasts.

Triple assessment of breast lumps To check out a lump, breast specialists take a "triple assessment" approach, using manual examination and mammography or ultrasound (see far left) and a procedure called fine-needle aspiration cytology (FNAC, see right). Since this approach is so thorough, false positives and false negatives are exceedingly rare.

Ruling out cancer Breast cancer is rare in women under 35 years of age, whatever the symptoms. If you're under 35, the odds are that your lump is a fibroadenoma. If you find a new – and the emphasis is on *new* – discrete lump, your doctor will always refer you to a hospital for assessment. The presence of a lump overrides any other symptom and you should expect your doctor to act accordingly, whether he or she believes the lump to be cancer or not. All doctors have the same priority – to exclude cancer.

The picture may be unclear if you already have some lumpiness in your breasts since this occasionally obscures a very small cancer. If you're under 35 and your other breast is also lumpy, however, cancer is unlikely – in fact, even if the lump is new, large, discrete and mobile, cancer is most improbable. If you're between 35 and 55, the lump is probably a cyst – this can be confirmed immediately with FNAC (see right). Cysts are uncommon in women over 55, when the risks of developing cancer increase.

Keeping the lump Excellent research has been done in Edinburgh, Scotland and Oxford, England, showing that most women with benign breast disorders are happy to forego surgery once they have been reassured that the condition is indeed benign. This is sensible and humane, especially since there is no connection between malignant change and most benign breast conditions. Because it's now possible to identify the vast majority of benign lumps without surgical removal, you have the right to keep your lump undisturbed. The only exception is a cyst where the simple procedure of FNAC will collapse and cure it. Most doctors will be happy to leave your lump untouched if:

• on examination, the lump feels smooth and is mobile;
• mammography or an ultrasound scan shows that the lump looks harmless;
• FNAC shows nothing untoward;
• follow-up examinations after three and six months show no change in the size or appearance of the lump. Although some doctors do not require follow-up examinations, you should always return if you notice any changes.

WHAT IS FNAC?

One of the three procedures in assessing a breast lump (see far left) is FNAC; the letters stand for Fine-Needle Aspiration Cytology. It is used to sample cells from the lump.

Under mammographic guidance, or ultrasound if the lump can't be felt, a fine needle is inserted into the lump.

If fluid is withdrawn, the lump is a cyst; the fluid can be aspirated (drawn off) and the cyst will disappear.

If the lump is solid, a sample of cells is removed and spread on a glass slide for staining (a smear) and microscopic examination.

FIBROADENOMAS AND CANCER

Fibroadenomas that are extremely large (that is, larger than a lemon) may undergo cancerous change at their centres. This kind of cancer grows slowly, does not spread to other parts of the body and does not kill.

The fact that some large fibroadenomas may become cancerous is therefore not a justification for removing all fibroadenomas, especially since this kind of change is rare. Having a fibroadenoma does not in itself increase your risk of developing cancer.

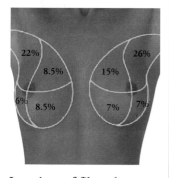

Locations of fibroadenomas
Although fibroadenomas can occur anywhere in the breast, they are often found near the nipple and are slightly more common in the left breast than in the right. No matter which breast they appear in, however, they are far more likely to occur in the upper outer quadrant and are seldom found in the lower ones. The picture shows the percentages found in each quadrant of either breast.

FIBROADENOMAS

These breast lumps are common in teenagers and women in their 20s (although they can occur at any age up to the menopause, or later if you're on HRT). They're simply over-developed lobules and are completely benign. You don't always need to have one removed, as long as you agree to further ultrasound and examination after six months. Most women opt for observation rather than removal.

Fibroadenomas can be very large – they vary from pea size to larger than a lemon. While they can grow anywhere in the breast, quite often they're found near the nipple. They feel smooth, firm and quite distinct, and move freely in your breast. Most doctors can recognize one simply by feeling it, but mammography or ultrasound and fine-needle aspiration cytology (see p. 33) or core needle biopsy (p. 58) will clinch the diagnosis.

Most women who get a fibroadenoma never get another one, but a few women have several over their lifetime. It is also possible to have more than one at a time or a single fibroadenoma involving more than one lobule. In extremely rare cases fibroadenomas may run in families.

Treatment options Once the diagnosis is confirmed, you can decide whether or not to have the lump removed (see p. 33). Most fibroadenomas come to nothing and shrink, so it's not unreasonable for your doctor to take a flexible attitude according to your age. If you're not worried, there's no need to have it removed. If you're under 25, cancer is so rare that a typical fibroadenoma can be left without risk, but you can have it removed if you wish. Fibroadenomas usually remain static, but if yours enlarges you can have it removed. Young women are often advised to watch and wait rather than undergo surgery and the resulting scarring. Where the picture is not clear, however, removal is wise.

Surgery is very simple and is done under local or general anaesthetic. To remove the lump, a small incision is made along the natural tension lines of the skin over it. The scars should be virtually invisible when they heal. Removal of a very large fibroadenoma can leave the breast misshapen, so discuss with your specialist the possibility of having your breast surgically refashioned, either in the same operation or later. This option will be available in most breast units. If not, the lump can be removed through an incision in the skin fold under the breast to give the best cosmetic result.

CYSTS

A cyst is a fluid-filled sac that is similar to a large blister buried in breast tissue. When you feel it you can usually detect its smooth outline and you may even be able to bounce it between two fingers as you push the fluid from side to side. This is particularly the case when the cyst is positioned near to the surface of the breast; when a cyst is buried deep in breast tissue, however, it will simply feel like a hard lump.

Quite often a cyst will seem to appear suddenly – even overnight. This is a very reassuring sign because anything that appears so suddenly is almost certainly harmless. Cysts are most commonly found in women in their 30s, 40s and 50s with the peak just prior to the menopause. It's possible, although rare, for cysts to occur in young women or in post-menopausal women.

Your doctor may be able to identify a lump as a cyst simply on physical examination, but most breast specialists will wish to confirm the diagnosis by following up with an ultrasound examination or a mammogram (mammography will detect a cyst but cannot distinguish between it and other breast lumps, however). Your doctor will then probably suggest fine-needle aspiration cytology (FNAC, see p. 33) as the next step to confirm the diagnosis.

Treatment With cysts, FNAC serves as both diagnosis and treatment in one. Aspiration can be done quickly, simply and painlessly as a routine procedure in the breast clinic. No local anaesthetic is necessary since all you will feel is a needle prick. The needle is pushed through the skin into the cyst and the fluid is aspirated into a syringe, causing the cyst to collapse and disappear. The whole procedure may be carried out under ultrasonic guidance, allowing you to watch as your doctor inserts the needle and aspirates the cyst and it disappears. Large cysts that are easily felt can be aspirated without the help of ultrasound.

The fluid from the cyst can be any colour – brown, yellow, greenish or milky white. (In breastfeeding women, a milk-filled cyst can form, and this is called a galactocele.) Studies have shown that there is no point in the aspirated fluid from the cyst being examined since the risk of cancer occurring in a cyst is so minute. If the fluid is evenly bloodstained, however, it will be sent to the laboratory for analysis of the sediment.

CYSTS AND CANCER

Cysts are rarely malignant, or not harmfully so. In a very few cases, a small cancer may grow inside the cyst, but it usually doesn't spread beyond the cyst into the surrounding breast tissue, and it cannot kill you.

If any evidence of cell growth is found in the cyst, your surgeon will operate on it.

If you have a simple cyst, you will not have any increased cancer risk.

Occasionally cysts reform. If this happens, you should return to your doctor to have the cyst aspirated (drained); although the cyst is harmless in itself, it could obscure other changes in the breasts.

A cyst that persistently refills after being drained carries a slightly increased risk of cancer.

Infection is the usual cause of periductal mastitis, which means inflammation around the milk ducts. Inflammation can also occur without infection; this form is thought to be due to irritation by stagnant secretions leaking from a dilated duct.

A bacterial infection may result in chronic inflammation of the milk ducts, and may cause the tissue behind the nipple to stand proud and be manifested as a lump – this is known as a granuloma.

Such an infection can be difficult to root out, even with antibiotics, so an abscess or a fistula (a seeping abscess with a permanent opening to the skin) may form. Whatever the cause of the mastitis, the end result is the same: gradual retraction of the nipple.

NIPPLE CONDITIONS

Benign disorders affecting the nipple are less common than lumpiness and pain, but can be equally worrying; like all breast complaints they warrant prompt diagnosis to eliminate a rare cancer and decide appropriate treatment.

DILATATION OF THE MILK DUCTS

The underlying change in the normal anatomy of the milk ducts as a woman grows older is called ectasia, or dilatation. Frequently this leads to blockage of the ducts with pooling of fluid behind the blockage. Infection may lead to chronic inflammation and sometimes an abscess forms.

Ectasia of the milk ducts occurs in the last part of the breast's development cycle. This condition is normal and may thus affect both breasts, but it should not usually cause change in the nipple. If an infection develops and affects the dilated ducts, surrounding inflammation (periductal mastitis, see left) can lead to the formation of scar tissue, which contracts and draws in the nipple. An infection that arises from ectasia is not normal, however. Fortunately, this complication hardly ever occurs except in women who smoke, and it won't heal if a woman continues to smoke.

The normal dilatation of the milk ducts with ageing, and inflammation or infection of the ducts, account for most nipple problems in women over 50, including recurrent subareolar abscesses (infected lumps) and nipple retraction. Occasionally ectasia causes breast pain.

NIPPLE DISCHARGE

Nipple discharge is far less common than pain and lumps, and is of no consequence when it appears only if the breast and nipple are squeezed. It's also normal for premenopausal women who have had children and for women who smoke to produce nipple secretions. The risk of cancer in a woman with nipple discharge is very low, especially if both breasts are involved. To establish the cause it's important to find out if the discharge is coming from one duct or several.

Diagnosis To evaluate nipple discharge, your doctor will perform a biopsy of the duct, also removing tissue under the nipple. Mammography often reveals the characteristic little needle-shaped deposits of calcium around and pointing towards the nipple. Surgical removal of the involved ducts may be suggested if the discharge is embarrassing.

If a lump is found in conjunction with nipple discharge, investigating it (see p. 32) takes priority. A lump beneath the areola in a breastfeeding woman is nearly always due to lactational mastitis (see below) complicated by an abscess.

Multiple duct discharge This is due to simple changes like ectasia and is nearly always benign. It is best left alone unless it's profuse and sufficient to stain clothes and cause embarrassment, but this is rare. Discharge caused by ectasia can be whitish, brown, grey or green, and watery or very thick. Surgical removal of the dilated or infected ducts won't be undertaken lightly; it can leave a woman unable to breastfeed and affect the sensation in the nipple and areola.

Occasionally, nipple discharge as a result of ectasia is accompanied by inflammation around the ducts, leaving the areolar skin red, hot and hard. If left untreated, this can lead to fistulae, although mostly in heavy smokers.

Single-duct discharge To doctors, discharge coming from a single duct is more significant than that from several ducts, but provided mammography shows no abnormality, surgery won't be required. Bloodstained discharge is usually due to a small benign papilloma (a wart-like growth) inside a duct, or to an ulcerated duct. The affected duct can be surgically removed. Rarely, a bloody discharge will be due to a ductal cancer; this doesn't have serious implications since this type of cancer is usually non-invasive (see p. 53).

NIPPLE INFECTIONS

The milk ducts are vulnerable to infection because bacteria can enter from the outside. Although such infections are unpleasant and often quite painful, they can be treated and are almost never a sign of something more sinister.

Lactational mastitis Nipple infections in a breastfeeding mother are the most common type. They nearly always arise from cracked, sore nipples; bacteria from the baby's mouth enters the lactiferous ducts through cracked skin and multiply rapidly in the milk. Occasionally, infection can result from a blocked duct. In both cases, the breast becomes tense, hot, reddened and painful.

Treatment Antibiotics combat the infection and analgesics deal with pain; neither should affect the baby. The breast should be rested for as short a time as possible because the baby's sucking keeps the milk flowing and this helps to overcome the infection; milk should be expressed in the meantime to keep the supply going. About one infection in

SUBAREOLAR INFECTIONS

Chronic infections of the breast around the areola usually affect women in their early thirties and are due to inflammation around the ducts. Smoking has been implicated as the most important cause, but how it damages the ducts isn't clear.

If the area is left untreated, it will become inflamed and an abscess may form. A mammary duct fistula is then a possibility if the abscess breaks down at the edge of the areola, and this can give rise to a permanent opening through the skin.

Antibiotics are the treatment of choice, but these infections are notoriously difficult to treat, especially if the patient goes on smoking. If the abscess fails to heal, an ultrasound scan will determine its extent and FNAC (see p. 33) will exclude an underlying cancer. The abscess can be drained but it may recur. A fistula must be surgically removed.

If the abscess is very large, or the nipple has become badly inverted, or infections recur even after removal of the fistula, larger-scale surgery may be recommended.

Surgery may be disfiguring, so seek a second opinion, especially if mastectomy is recommended. Most women are happy with major duct excision if they're forewarned of the consequences such as lopsided breasts and loss of nipple sensation.

PAGET'S DISEASE

Although it looks like eczema, Paget's disease is actually a form of very slow-growing cancer, and tends to be associated with its in situ form (see p. 53). It's therefore not a benign condition but is mentioned here because it is important to consider Paget's disease whenever eczema of the nipple occurs (see right).

Paget's disease can sometimes be distinguished from eczema just by looking: it invariably starts on the nipple as a non-scaly, moist and erosive patch with a florid, raw, red surface, a definite outline and profuse discharge. Generally only one nipple is affected; it is rare for it to affect both nipples.

Another distinguishing characteristic of Paget's disease is that it develops slowly and is persistent – it won't clear up spontaneously and then recur like eczema. If Paget's disease is suspected, your doctor will recommend a biopsy and perhaps a mammogram.

ten goes on to form an abscess, which must be drained in hospital, under general anaesthetic if necessary. Once this has been done and the pain has subsided, you can breastfeed again. Sometimes ultrasound will show a small abscess, which can be treated by drawing out the pus with a needle.

Non-lactational mastitis Nipple infections are very rare if you are not breastfeeding. Women with lowered immunity, diabetes or who have had breast surgery are most at risk.

SKIN CONDITIONS

The skin of the breasts is thin and sensitive but need not be more prone to problems than skin elsewhere on the body provided proper care is taken (see p. 12).

Cracked nipples During breastfeeding, the skin around the nipples is exposed to milk and vigorous sucking, both of which can damage the skin. Prevention is the best approach: the nipples should be gently dabbed clean after each feed and a baby who is properly latched on will not need to suck hard to feed well. Applying a drop of baby lotion to your breast pad can also help. If the nipples do become cracked, it's important to get advice on positioning the baby correctly on the breast and taking her off. This is best done by pushing down gently on the baby's chin to break the airtight seal between her mouth and the nipple. Treatment for cracked nipples must be prompt, since they are vulnerable to infections (see p. 37).

Eczema Classically, eczema starts on the areolar skin and later spreads to the nipple; it usually appears on both nipples and can be localized or associated with generalized eczema elsewhere on the body. It develops quite quickly and may clear up but then recur. The involved skin is usually scaly, red, itchy and moist and the patch of eczema is likely to have an irregular outline. Eczema will normally respond to one percent hydrocortisone cream.

Areolar gland disorders There are three kinds of gland in the areolar skin and all of them can lead to problems. The apocrine sweat glands can become infected and form cysts; the sebaceous glands can also form cysts; and the accessory mammary glands can discharge or become infected.

Treatment Infection of the sweat glands can usually be cleared with an antibiotic cream, but the glands very often have to be removed if the infection persists. Cysts can be removed under local anaesthetic if they are troublesome. Discharge and infection usually respond to antibiotics.

BREAST CANCER

Understanding the causes and effects of a disease such as breast cancer can greatly improve your chances of avoiding and defeating it. Knowledge of risk and preventive factors can help you to reduce your own risk of getting breast cancer. This includes making both life choices – such as having your first baby before 30 years of age and breastfeeding – and lifestyle changes, such as keeping your weight down and your consumption of alcohol low. Early detection and diagnosis play an important role in the successful treatment of breast cancer, and in the prognosis and long-term outlook. Modern techniques of grading and staging mean that doctors can tailor treatment to the particular needs of each patient.

AIDS AND BREAST CANCER

Women who are HIV positive or who have AIDS do not appear to have a higher risk of developing breast cancer than the average woman.

This interesting finding contradicts a popular belief: that weakening of the immune system – whether by disease or by stressful experiences – gives cancerous cells more chance to take hold in the body, and so contributes to the development of breast cancer.

UNDERSTANDING BREAST CANCER

Cancer of the breast need not be fatal. Only one breast lump in about eight turns out to be cancerous and, of those that do, a considerable number are of the non-invasive type – that is, they do not spread beyond their place of origin and therefore cannot kill. A cancer that is less than 1 centimetre (½ inch) in diameter is still at a very early stage; there is therefore only a small chance that it has spread and less risk of its being fatal. One of the main aims of this chapter, therefore, is to curb the panic that may grip you when you discover a lump, so that you seek advice immediately and give yourself the best chance, rather than succumb to the paralysing fear that the prospect of cancer may bring.

The psychological reactions to finding a lump and being given a diagnosis of cancer are complex. Breast cancer has social, emotional and sexual consequences that will affect not only a woman's health but her relationships, her lifestyle and her body image. A knowledgeable and well-informed woman is best placed to take an active role in her treatment, and to cultivate the positive state of mind that can contribute to the defeat of the disease.

It's important for you to know that, even when a diagnosis of breast cancer is made, there are different types. Not all cancers have the same degree of invasiveness or potential for spread, so not all have a poor outlook. A positive attitude is a real asset, possibly as vital as some medical treatments.

THE NATURE OF BREAST CANCER

Breast cancer is a family of conditions, not a single entity. The common feature of every type, however, is that certain cells start to grow out of control. Cell growth is normally restricted to simple repair so that an organ is kept up to scratch; it is held in check by chemicals that ensure growth is orderly and never gets out of hand. Cancer starts when the brakes on growth are taken off, or when they are no longer effective, or when cells become insensitive to them. Cell growth then becomes uncontrolled and disorderly and the cells themselves may start to look abnormal. Because cell growth is rapid in a cancer, it absorbs a great deal of body energy. This is why cancer is often accompanied by weight loss, although this is rare in breast cancer.

Tumours and spread The word tumour simply means a lump. Most tumours are not cancerous. They are usually benign; the growth of cells is confined to the area where the tumour starts. Tumours whose cells don't spread to other parts of the body are not fatal. In contrast, the cells that make up cancerous tumours are invasive. They spread beyond their original location, not just into adjacent tissues, but to other distant parts of the body, and as they invade tissue they destroy it.

The original tumour is known as the primary. Tumours that arise from these cancerous cells that have spread elsewhere are called secondaries or metastases. To determine how aggressive cancer cells are and how far they have spread, if at all, grading and staging tests (see pp. 60–61) are done. These tests also serve as a basis for deciding on treatment.

Spread through the lymphatic system Cancers of the breast often spread first into the lymph nodes in the armpits (the axillary lymph nodes), causing swelling. They may also spread to lymph nodes under the breastbone and above the collarbone. (This is why you should always check your armpits and collarbone for swollen lymph nodes whenever you do your regular breast self-examination.)

Cancer in the bloodstream While the first sign of spread may be enlarged lymph nodes, spread via the bloodstream is probably more important in determining the final outcome of the disease. The most recent research suggests that breast-cancer cells, or particles of them ("seeds"), enter the bloodstream relatively early in the course of the disease. This is why modern treatments, like chemotherapy, are aimed at eradicating cancer cells from the body *as a whole* rather than just dealing with the tumour locally.

PUTTING BREAST CANCER IN PERSPECTIVE

• Breast cancer, over a lifetime, affects 1 in 12 women and causes around 15,000 deaths a year in the UK.

• Five times more women suffer from the disease than die from it. In a given year, of 100,000 women who live with breast cancer, 80,000 do not die.

• More than 70 percent of women who have operable disease will be alive and well five years after the diagnosis.

• By the age of 50, your chances of dying from breast cancer will have dropped dramatically from 12 in 70 to 1 in 70, and the odds get better with every year you live after that without developing it (continued p. 42).

FIBROBLASTS

Some research has centred on whether there may be a link between the character of a woman's breast tissue and her risk of getting breast cancer.

Researchers now suggest that it may not be the glandular elements of the breast that determine whether cells change from normal to cancerous, but cells called fibroblasts.

Fibroblasts lie among the fat and connective tissue of the breast and produce a number of chemical messengers called growth factors. These seem to communicate with breast cancer cells, stimulating their growth and ability to spread.

Cancer cells need a rich blood supply to support their rapid growth, and fibroblasts appear to encourage the formation of new blood vessels in tissues surrounding the cancer that provide the necessary blood.

It's probable that fibroblasts in some women are more likely to support the growth of cancer cells than fibroblasts in other women. This finding may help in part to explain why some breast cancers are hereditary.

Fatal diseases
This chart shows that stroke and heart disease cause many more deaths than breast cancer among women of all ages in the developed world.

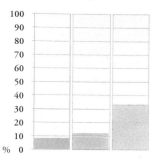

KEY

	DEATHS FROM BREAST CANCER
	DEATHS FROM STROKE
	DEATHS FROM HEART DISEASE

Your chances of dying from something else
Breast cancer (represented on the graph by the green area) is the most common cause of death in women between 35 and 55. While it is more common in women over 55, it is less likely to be the cause of death in this age group.

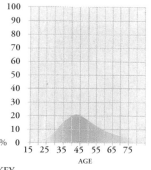

KEY

| | DEATHS FROM OTHER CAUSES |
| | DEATHS FROM BREAST CANCER |

• In statistical terms, breast cancer accounts for almost one in five of all new cancer cases among women.
• In women between 35 and 55, it ranks as the commonest cause of death overall, *but*
  – for every breast lump found to be cancerous, about eight others will be benign and therefore harmless;
  – even with cancerous lumps, six or seven out of ten will be treated without removing the breast;
  – if the lump is diagnosed and treated early, you'll be one of the 85 percent of women who survive at least five years;
  – in post-menopausal women, deaths from breast cancer pale into insignificance when compared with the number of deaths caused by heart disease;
  – by the time you are in your mid-60s, your chances of dying from breast cancer (as opposed to dying from a condition such as heart disease) are probably less than half what they were when you were 50.
• So, although the chances of getting breast cancer increase as women age, the chances of dying from it become less with each successive year that they live.

THE GENETICS OF CANCER

A healthy cell has a well-defined shape. It is a responsible "team player", multiplying only when the balance of signals is favourable. Built into cell growth, however, is the hazard of genetic mutations, or random changes. Then, the cell becomes damaged; it may appear normal, but it is slightly less responsive to external signals. As genetic damage accumulates, a cell can become deaf to external messages that inhibit growth and start to show signs of malignancy. In particular, it loses its regular shape and outline and multiplies uncontrollably. Cancer probably develops because cells suffer irreversible damage to their genes. Events that cause damage to genes are called trigger factors and those that facilitate cell growth are called promoters.

The development of a cancer cell takes time, even several lifetimes. On the other hand, it can take as little as ten years depending on how damaged the genes were when they passed from parent to child. Severely damaged genes may respond quickly to an environmental trigger, such as prolonged exposure to menstrual cycling (see right) in the case of breast cancer. Two breast cancer genes have been identified: BRCA1 and BRCA2 (see p. 50), but there are likely to be many more.

RISK AND PROTECTIVE FACTORS

Some women are more likely to get cancer of the breast than others: the risk can be connected with geographic location, particular cultures, specific personal traits and lifestyle features. Some women inherit a susceptibility to the disease, which then requires one or more environmental risk factors in order that breast cancer should develop. Genetic factors therefore interact with environmental factors, but unfortunately doctors don't know how.

Doctors do know enough, however, to help them to identify women who are at high risk. This in turn promotes early detection of breast cancer and enables some women to change their lifestyles and make life choices to reduce their risk. Try to take a positive attitude and remember that some risk factors can be turned upside-down to become protective factors: if having your first baby late increases the risk, you might consider having an early first child to lower your risk (see Protection in pregnancy, p. 44).

Hormones The patterns of a woman's hormones and their fluctuations during menstruation, pregnancy and lactation all play an important part in determining her risk of developing breast cancer. Hormones from other sources, such as the contraceptive pill and hormone replacement therapy, may have an effect, although this is much less.

Menstruation The risk of breast cancer appears to be increased both by an early onset of menstruation, medically termed menarche, and by a late cessation of menstruation, which is called menopause. In the developed world, the average age at which a woman starts to menstruate seems to be getting earlier, and the average age at menopause getting later, and this lengthening of "menstrual life" could be a contributory factor in the apparent increase in breast-cancer rates (see column, p. 44).

Researchers are coming to believe that the *total number of menstrual cycles* in a woman's lifetime determines her cancer risk. The number of menstrual cycles before the first pregnancy may be even more important, however. It is possible that the breasts are more sensitive to the action of hormones before they have fully developed – that is, before they have produced milk – and this would explain why age at first pregnancy is so important (continued p. 44).

TYPES OF RISK

There are two different ways of describing risk: relative risk and absolute risk.

Relative risk describes how a single factor may increase risk. Take the risk factor of having a family history of breast cancer. The relative risk of a woman whose mother had breast cancer is 2, meaning that she is twice as likely to get the disease as a woman with no family history of breast cancer.

Absolute risk is more precise, and denotes the number of likely cases of breast cancer in a specific number of women over a given time. The absolute risk of breast cancer, however, is 1 woman per 1,000 per year; this means that one woman in one thousand will get breast cancer in a year. For women with a family history of breast cancer, therefore, the absolute risk is 2 per 1,000 per year.

MENSTRUAL LIFE AND RISK

Your "menstrual life" links three important risk factors for breast cancer – age at first period, age at menopause and number of pregnancies – that determine your total exposure to oestrogen. The longer the exposure, the greater the risk. Even quite small differences between women can add up to significant differences in overall risk, as the following two examples show.

Liz

Age at menopause	*48*
Less age at first period	*–14*
Less time spent pregnant (years)	*–3*
Total years' exposure to oestrogen	**31**

Joan

Age at menopause	*52*
Less age at first period	*–12*
Less time spent pregnant (years)	*–1½*
Total years' exposure to oestrogen	**38½**

It is also possible that a fertile lifetime of menstruation is, in biological terms, an abnormal state for the human female and so predisposes women to develop breast cancer. It's only relatively recently that women stopped spending a great proportion of their reproductive life either pregnant or breastfeeding, and it's only in the twentieth century that women in any numbers have lived long enough to reach the menopause at all. The average girl in the developed world now starts to menstruate before the age of 12, but will then wait until she is 27 or 28 years old to have her first baby, exposing her to almost 16 years of continuous menstrual cycling before her first pregnancy. This doesn't happen in many other cultures. An African girl may not start menstruating until she's 17 or 18 because she's undernourished, and may then become pregnant almost at once, saving her from years of exposure to cyclical oestrogens.

Protection in pregnancy Having babies undoubtedly protects women against breast cancer; this may be because it saves a woman from being exposed to cyclical oestrogens for nine months. The major protection seems to be conferred by the first pregnancy, which must be carried to term to be protective; a first pregnancy that ends in abortion or miscarriage does not have any protective effect.

Not having children and having a first baby late in life both seem to increase the chances of developing breast cancer. For women who have their first child after the age of 30, the risk of breast cancer is about twice that of women who have their first child before the age of 20. Women who remain childless are at increased risk, and this may partly explain why infertility in older women is linked to breast cancer. Surprisingly, women who have their first child after the age of 35 appear to be at an even higher risk than women who have no children.

The contraceptive pill The oral contraceptive pill was introduced 30 years ago and has been used by about 150 million women. Huge long-term research studies have not uncovered any *substantial* increased risk of breast cancer in women who take the pill. Breast cancer is fairly common, as is the practice of taking the pill, so if breast cancer develops in a woman who is on the pill, it can't be assumed that the two are related; it might have happened anyway.

Against these very small increases in risk, doctors have to weigh the fact that the pill has a protective effect against ovarian cancer. For a woman at risk of ovarian cancer, this protective effect would outweigh the breast cancer risk. Some studies have shown a reduction in benign breast disease among contraceptive pill users, which could reduce the risk of breast cancer.

Hormone replacement therapy Menopausal symptoms have been successfully treated with hormone replacement therapy (HRT) for more than 50 years. There has been no dramatic increase in breast cancer, however, since the use of HRT became fairly widespread some two decades ago, suggesting that any risk is very small. Most researchers in this field agree that in the first ten years of use there is no increased risk associated with HRT. After that time there may be a very small increased risk, but for the average healthy woman, it would appear that the use of HRT does not increase breast-cancer risk any more than having a first baby after the age of 30.

As with the contraceptive pill, there are also benefits to be weighed against any possible risk. HRT has a protective effect against cancers of the lung, colon, ovary and cervix. It also protects against osteoporosis. Women on HRT who develop breast cancer usually have a less invasive form of cancer and are more likely to respond to hormone treatment. Women who develop breast cancer after having taken HRT for eight years have an improved survival rate Finally, women who have used HRT seem to have a lower mortality rate at any age from any cause than those who have not.

Even for women who have had breast cancer, HRT needn't be ruled out as long as there is careful follow-up from a doctor who is expert in this field. If you fall into this category, you should talk it over with a gynaecologist as well as a cancer specialist.

Family history A family history of breast cancer is a strong risk factor in itself and makes all other risk factors potentially more significant. The increase in risk depends on how close the relative is and on how many relatives have had breast cancer. The risk is greater if the affected relative developed breast cancer under the age of 50, and increases still further if *two* female relatives are affected. The risk is greatest if your mother developed breast cancer under the age of 35.

A woman whose mother developed cancer in both breasts before the age of 35, for instance, has a 50 percent chance of developing breast cancer herself. This familial susceptibility to breast cancer is now known to be related

Family history and risk
The more relatives a woman has with breast cancer, and the younger they are when they develop the disease, the higher her own risk becomes.

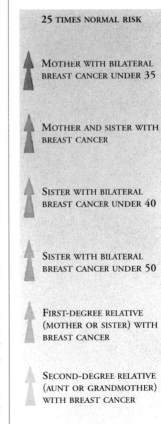

25 TIMES NORMAL RISK

MOTHER WITH BILATERAL BREAST CANCER UNDER 35

MOTHER AND SISTER WITH BREAST CANCER

SISTER WITH BILATERAL BREAST CANCER UNDER 40

SISTER WITH BILATERAL BREAST CANCER UNDER 50

FIRST-DEGREE RELATIVE (MOTHER OR SISTER) WITH BREAST CANCER

SECOND-DEGREE RELATIVE (AUNT OR GRANDMOTHER) WITH BREAST CANCER

NORMAL RISK

BREAST CANCER "LEAGUE TABLE"

The following list shows the relative positions of 24 countries in a "league table" of breast cancer rates, with countries in Western Europe at the top of the league.

1 England and Wales
2 Denmark
3 Scotland
4 Northern Ireland
5 Netherlands
6 Belgium
7 Switzerland
8 New Zealand
9 Canada
10 Germany
11 United States
12 Hungary
13 Czech Republic and Slovakia
14 Australia
15 Argentina
16 France
17 Norway
18 Sweden
19 Portugal
20 Poland
21 Bulgaria
22 Greece
23 Hong Kong
24 Japan

to two genes, labelled BRCA1 and BRCA2 (see p. 50). Being born into a "breast-cancer family" (see pp. 49–50) carries the greatest risk, and it's important to identify these women who are at high risk of developing breast cancer.

Age Given that environmental factors can react with a genetic predisposition to trigger the growth of breast cancer, it stands to reason that the longer a woman lives the more likely she is to be exposed to these environmental triggers and the higher her risk is of developing breast cancer. This supposition is borne out by the statistics: about half of all breast cancers occur in women aged 50–64, with a further 30 percent in women aged over 70. This means that 80 percent of breast cancers occur over the age of 50.

Geography Although the frequency of breast cancer varies widely throughout the world (see left) the disease seems to single out white women living in colder climates in highly industrialized societies, and it's the lifestyle of the developed world that is largely to blame. Women from low-risk areas (for instance Japan, which has one of the lowest rates of breast cancer in the entire world) who move to and settle permanently in higher-risk countries, such as the US, climb into a higher risk group for breast cancer. Environmental factors therefore seem to be stronger than racial or inherited ones. There is even evidence that shows rates of breast cancer increasing as countries become more industrialized.

Radiation Doctors have known for some time that high doses of radiation can promote the development of breast cancer. In the past, women who received high-dose chest X-rays to check on treatment for tuberculosis ran an increased risk of developing cancer. Japanese women who were exposed to enormously high doses of radiation from the atomic bombs at Hiroshima and Nagasaki are still developing breast cancer at higher rates than other Japanese women of the same age living in other parts of Japan.

Protection in breastfeeding Breastfeeding does seem to protect against breast cancer, although pregnancy is even more important; an early pregnancy (see p. 44) is protective regardless of whether a woman breastfeeds or bottlefeeds. Some evidence from UK studies suggests that breastfeeding even for a very short time is protective. Since breastfeeding has so substantial a protective effect, and since it is available to all women who give birth, it's astonishing that more women don't do it. I would urge all women to consider breastfeeding, even for as short a time as a couple of weeks.

Diet The Western diet is constantly cited as a risk factor for breast cancer, but the evidence is pretty thin. The original connection came from an observation that dietary fat can cause breast tumours in rats. Such evidence can't be directly applied to human beings, but it was an interesting lead. Studies of total fat intake, however, have not found that women with breast cancer consume a significantly higher amount of fat than women without; the relationship may reflect total intake of calories rather than fat intake alone. Breast cancer risk seems more influenced by obesity than by fat consumption.

People who eat a diet high in fat tend to eat less fruit and vegetables, so it could be that the risk is due to a deficiency of fibre rather than an excess of fat. Quite recent evidence suggests that a diet rich in cereals and vegetables may protect against breast cancer. Fibre is thought to influence oestrogen metabolism and some vitamin derivatives may have a protective effect, particularly vitamin E and beta-carotene, which is a form of vitamin A.

A study from Cambridge, England, has shown that a soya-rich diet will lengthen the menstrual cycle by two or three days. Over a lifetime this would mean significantly fewer cycles, having a beneficial effect with regard to breast cancer (see p. 44). The active components of soya are isoflavones, which have a strong oestrogenic effect.

Obesity Women who are overweight have a higher risk of dying from breast cancer than their leaner sisters. The pattern of obesity seems to be important in defining cancer risk. When fat is concentrated around the trunk, giving a ratio between waist and hip measurements of greater than one (an "apple shape"), cancer risk is higher than in women who retain a well-defined waist with bigger hips ("pear shapes"). This pattern of obesity is linked with a number of diseases, such as heart disease in men. It's a common fat distribution among post-menopausal and infertile women, in whom breast cancer rates are higher than average.

Alcohol Excessive alcohol intake increases a woman's risk of developing breast cancer in the long term, since alcohol can interfere with the body's metabolism of oestrogen. Both alcohol and oestrogen are broken down in the liver and, after many years of exposure to alcohol, the liver loses its ability to metabolize oestrogen. This results in increased levels of oestrogen in the blood, a factor known to increase the risk of breast cancer (continued p. 48).

SMOKING

Rates of breast cancer are lower in smokers than in non-smokers. This can never be advocated as a reason for smoking, however, since the risk of dying from a smoking-related disease such as lung cancer far outweighs that of dying from breast cancer.

It is thought that smoking exerts an anti-oestrogenic effect, accelerating the onset of the menopause; smokers typically reach the menopause three to four years earlier than women who do not smoke.

Smokers tend to be thinner than those who don't smoke; it is known that oestrogens are manufactured in the fatty tissues and that obesity is a risk factor for breast cancer (see left). Smokers also have less benign breast disease than non-smokers and this could partly explain the reduced risk.

The protective effect that smoking confers is greater among post-menopausal than pre-menopausal women, and seems to operate only as long as you go on smoking. When you stop, the protection is lost.

As yet, doctors don't fully understand why smoking has an anti-oestrogenic effect. One study has found that women who smoke have higher levels of male sex hormones, such as testosterone, which has anti-oestrogenic properties.

This link with alcohol is not a great risk and must be kept in perspective. If one thousand women over the age of 30 drank moderately for two years, there would be one extra case of breast cancer among them.

WHAT YOU CAN DO

Although you can't control factors like your family history or age at menopause, you can change some aspects of your lifestyle to make a difference to your risk of breast cancer.
- Restrict red meat and fat in your diet and increase your fibre intake by eating plenty of wholegrain cereals and at least five portions of fruit and vegetables every day.
- Enjoy alcohol only in moderation.
- Keep your body fat down by eating a balanced diet and taking regular exercise.
- Plan to have your first baby by the age of 30.
- If you have babies, breastfeed – the longer the better.

Comparison of risk
The chart below looks at the different factors that can affect your risk of developing breast cancer and helps you to compare them. Remember that the lowest possible risk has a score of 1.0.

FACTORS THAT CAN AFFECT THE RISK OF DEVELOPING BREAST CANCER

RISK FACTOR	LOWEST RISK		SLIGHT INCREASE		MODERATE INCREASE	
AGE AT FIRST MENSTRUAL PERIOD	16 years (late)	1.0	15 years (late) 11–14 years	1.1 1.3		
AGE AT MENOPAUSE	Before 45	1.0	45–54	1.4	Over 55	2.1
AGE AT BIRTH OF FIRST CHILD	Before 20	1.0	20–29	1.45	Over 30 years or no children	1.9
FAMILY HISTORY	None	1.0	Mother affected before age 60 Mother affected after age 60	2.0 1.4	Two first-degree relatives affected (i.e., mother and sister)	4.0–6.0
BENIGN BREAST DISEASE	None	1.0	Increase in number of cells	2.0	Atypical hyperplasia (see p. 53)	4.5
ALCOHOL INTAKE	None	1.0	1 drink a day 2 drinks a day	1.4 1.7	3 drinks a day	2.0
RADIATION EXPOSURE	No special exposure	1.0	Repeated X-rays	1.5–2.0	Atomic bomb	3.0
ORAL CONTRACEPTIVES	Never used or no longer used	1.0	Currently used	1.5	Prolonged use before pregnancy	2.0
HRT	Never used or no longer used	1.0	Currently used all ages	1.4	Used longer than ten years or currently used over 60	2.1

BREAST-CANCER FAMILIES

A single first-degree relative (that is, mother or sister) with breast cancer doubles anyone's risk of cancer, but in breast-cancer families the risks are even greater. A breast-cancer family is one in which the risk of a woman developing breast cancer is determined almost totally by family history, and appears to be independent of other risk factors, except atypical hyperplasia (see p. 53).

Breast-cancer families, although quite rare, have been studied for more than two millennia and were first reported in Roman medical literature of AD 100. In the 1860s, an American doctor, Paul Broca, described many instances of breast cancer in combination with bowel cancer in several generations of his wife's family. He was describing what we now call hereditary breast cancer (HBC). The word hereditary means that the cancer runs through a family affecting successive generations of women. The pattern of inheritance nearly always suggests that the hereditary factor is extremely strong. The factor responsible has been narrowed down to one or two genes (see p. 50), and since it's so strong, it is known as a dominant gene. Although hereditary breast cancer puts women at very high risk, it accounts for only a small proportion of all cases of breast cancer – between five and ten percent.

A rigorous approach There are several important features of HBC that profoundly affect treatment. The first is the early age of onset. Breast cancer is more common in older women as a rule, with an average age of 62 years among women affected, but in breast-cancer families the average age is 44. Second, there is often more than one tumour in the breast. Finally, the cancer may affect both breasts.

These three characteristics have an enormous bearing on how doctors view familial breast cancer. Women in these families need to be identified, and made aware that they are in danger of developing breast cancer early, and in both breasts. Any woman who is aware of her risk should seek advice from a breast unit while still in her teens or early 20s. Because of the aggressive nature of this cancer, doctors are more likely to be receptive to the idea of prophylactic (preventive) mastectomy (see p. 51) together with breast reconstruction (see pp. 84–85), although medically such a radical course is hard to justify when inheritance of the gene cannot yet be conclusively proved (continued p. 50).

The shadow cast by the hereditary aspect of HBC falls on all aspects of managing it. Monitoring of the health of the breasts must be rigorous and scrupulous. It must include regular check-ups, mammograms, ultrasound scans where appropriate and biopsies of any suspicious changes.

Identifying women at risk At present, the most important tool for doctor and patient is a thorough family history. There's unfortunately no way of testing for the precise genes and chromosomes associated with HBC and identifying vulnerable women before the cancer appears, although there is hope that such tests will become possible in the next few years. Until then, a careful family pedigree and close surveillance, together with frequent physical examinations and mammograms, are the best defence. Much controversy surrounds the age for starting mammographic screening. The problem with mammograms in younger women is that their breasts are more dense than those of older women and cancers are difficult to pick up. Several studies have shown, however, that early detection is possible, and it is certainly worthwhile in breast-cancer families.

Careful surveillance of cancer families is essential. This is best done by gathering the female members of the family together to explain how cancers can run through each generation in a family, offering counselling and ensuring that each woman is vigorously screened and tested in order to detect any cancers as early as possible.

Breast cancer genes Two of the genes that are responsible for inherited breast cancer were finally identified in 1994, and it is likely that there are more to be found. These two, called BRCA1 and BRCA2, are probably responsible for more than half the cases of hereditary breast cancer. A woman carrying either of them has about an 80 percent risk of contracting breast cancer during her lifetime, and a 70 percent risk after the age of 50. The genes can be passed on by either parent (not just the mother), and there is a 50–50 chance that children will inherit them.

At the moment, no gene test is available (there are many possible gene mutations, presenting complex problems for testing), but it is probable that within the next three years, women from breast-cancer families could be offered a test. Women found to carry the genes would then have the options of increased monitoring to detect cancer early on, including annual mammography from age 35, tamoxifen therapy, or prophylactic (preventive) mastectomy.

PREVENTIVE MEASURES

An overview of breast-cancer risk factors (see pp. 43–48) shows there are some that can be controlled to reduce risk, notably diet, alcohol intake, an early first child and – for women who have children – breastfeeding. For women at very high risk, however, some kind of prevention in the form of hormone treatment or surgery may be advisable.

Tamoxifen A complex drug with both oestrogenic and anti-oestrogenic properties, tamoxifen was first used in the treatment of breast cancer and is now being studied as a way of preventing it among high-risk women, particularly those with a strong family history where breast cancer may appear at an early age (see pp. 49–50). Tamoxifen is used to treat women who already have breast cancer; not only does it reduce the risk of recurrence and improve mortality rates, but in the long term it also reduces by half the risk of getting cancer in the other breast, a cause for great concern for women with a family history of breast cancer.

Just as fibroblast growth factors (see p. 41) promote breast cancer, other growth factors suppress it. The production of suppressor growth factors is stimulated by tamoxifen, and this is one of the reasons why it could be effective in the prevention of breast cancer.

Because of its action on the production of the hormone, oestrogen, tamoxifen has side-effects when taken for long periods, causing menopausal symptoms and an early onset of the menopause. One study has raised the possibility of a slightly increased risk of uterine cancer; others do not. This is being studied to see if any risk actually exists. Tamoxifen has life-saving properties other than reducing the risk of breast cancer, however. It seems to protect against heart attacks – in a recent study in Scotland it led to a significant reduction in deaths from heart disease – and osteoporosis (brittle bones caused by loss of bone protein).

Prophylactic (preventive) mastectomy If you are at high risk of developing breast cancer, you may have seen your mother or sister die from the disease, and may consider mastectomy as an effective way to prevent it in yourself. Prophylactic mastectomy aims to reduce the risk of breast cancer by removing as much breast tissue as possible. Reconstruction may be carried out to rebuild the breast. In such a case, you do not have the option of a subcutaneous mastectomy, which is an operation where the breast tissue

MAKING THE DECISION: PROS

You should consider both the pros and the cons (see p. 52) if you are thinking about prophylactic mastectomy.

- *There is no definite evidence to prove that prophylactic mastectomy reduces a woman's chance of getting cancer, but it probably does, as long as the operation is a total mastectomy.*

- *The operation certainly reduces painful symptoms and tender lumpiness in the breast as part of the menstrual cycle, although mastalgia (breast pain) alone would never be a reason for mastectomy.*

- *For women who cannot live normal lives for fear of breast cancer, it can provide a new lease of life.*

- *Modern surgical procedures mean that the breasts can be reconstructed (see pp. 84–85).*

MAKING THE DECISION: CONS

Reconstruction may be done to rebuild the breasts after prophylactic mastectomy. You should consider the risks of this operation as well.

- *General anaesthesia is a risk in its own right.*

- *There may be complications including bleeding, infection, skin loss, nipple loss and damage to the implant.*

- *Capsular contraction may occur, where the capsule of scar tissue that forms around the implant contracts and becomes as hard as wood. Massaging the breasts may reduce the firmness, but if they are very hard, treatment can be quite complicated and may involve further surgery.*

- *Complications can occur if an abdominal flap is used for reconstruction (see pp. 84–85).*

- *The reconstructed breast is rarely as attractive as the original breast, and there may be permanent scarring and loss of sensation.*

- *More than one operation may be needed to achieve the best results or manage complications.*

- *There's no guarantee that cancer will be prevented: not all breast tissue is removed and any that is left behind is still a potential site for breast cancer.*

is removed from beneath the skin and an implant inserted, leaving the nipple and areola intact. The operation *must* be a total mastectomy; anything else is not justifiable. If your doctor should suggest a subcutaneous mastectomy, question its reliability and usefulness and get a second opinion.

Prophylactic mastectomy, in which one or both breasts are removed, is a controversial operation. Many doctors are loath to remove healthy breast tissue when cancer may never develop. Also crucial is whether the operation is effective enough in preventing breast cancer when powerful, non-surgical treatments, such as tamoxifen therapy (see p. 51), could accomplish the same goal. When contemplating prophylactic mastectomy, you must remember that there is no guarantee that breast cancer will be prevented. For these reasons, you will be considered eligible to have both breasts removed only if you fulfil the following strict criteria:
- an unarguable family history and an estimated 50 percent chance of getting breast cancer;
- your clear understanding that you have a 50–50 chance of inheriting the high-risk gene, so that you have an equal chance of carrying and not carrying the gene (the latter would mean you are at normal risk for breast cancer);
- the presence of additional factors that would raise the risk above 50 percent, such as two sisters being affected or atypical hyperplasia (see column, p. 53).

Other factors that would also be taken into consideration are breasts that are difficult to examine both clinically and radiographically, and severe cancer phobia. You should decide to have prophylactic mastectomy only after careful discussion of your precise risk, details of the operation and the likely outcome with a specialist breast surgeon and the other members of the breast management team. Even better would be counselling by two surgeons who can evaluate your particular risk factors and their implications. Finally, you should also consult close family and friends. Most women, when advised that they have a chance of not carrying the high-risk gene, opt for intensive follow-up screening and testing rather than surgery.

The majority of women at high risk are monitored most effectively by breast self-examination and regular physical examinations and mammograms. In addition, fine-needle aspiration cytology (see column, p. 33) is decreasing the need for open biopsy if a breast lump should occur, and biopsy is available for any suspicious breast areas that may arise.

NON-INVASIVE CANCER

The glands and ducts that make up the breast lobules are in a state of growth, development and shrinkage during a woman's fertile life. Overgrowth of cells or hyperplasia, as it is called, may occur in any part of the lobes or ducts. The word hyperplasia without qualification always implies a benign condition, although it carries a small increase in the risk of cancer. In some hyperplasias, however, the cells become somewhat unusual or atypical. This is referred to as atypical hyperplasia, and has a moderate chance of turning into a localized cancer. (A woman with a family history of breast cancer who develops atypical hyperplasia moves into a very high-risk group indeed.)

Actual cancer comes at the far end of the hyperplasia spectrum, but, at first at least, it is the non-invasive "cancer in situ" (*in situ* means that the cancer is confined to its place of origin). This term is used for patterns of cell growth that are confined to the duct or lobule where they originated, but carry a high risk of becoming invasive (see right).

PRE-INVASIVE DISEASE

As cell growth proceeds from hyperplasia, which is benign, towards malignancy, it reaches an in-between stage – cancer "in situ". This is a crucial distinction to make, since these cancers by definition are not invasive and they are seldom fatal. There are two kinds: ductal carcinoma in situ (DCIS) and lobular carcinoma in situ (LCIS).

In situ carcinomas are confined to the duct or lobule in which they start growing, and rarely invade the surrounding breast. A true lump is often difficult to detect and, unless there is some other symptom such as nipple discharge, the majority of these lumps are picked up only through screening mammograms, when the characteristic tiny Y-shaped calcifications of DCIS are seen.

In situ cancers sometimes pose a problem for treatment because it is not known how many may progress to invasive cancer, nor how long they may take to do so. Nor has one approach to the treatment of DCIS and LCIS been proved to be substantially better than any other.

Because of the risk that an invasive cancer may develop, preventive mastectomy may be an option. Most doctors, however, would probably adopt the compromise of a wide excision to remove the cancerous tissue and a watch-policy,

UNDERSTANDING HYPERPLASIA

Hyperplasia (cell overgrowth) has four stages. The stage that most concerns doctors is the second: atypical hyperplasia (see below). When assessing hyperplasia, there are several features that doctors look at to decide whether the condition is benign or whether there is a risk of cancer.

- *Deciding features include the rate at which the cells are dividing; the way the cells are organized; and the features of the cells themselves.*

- *In normal circumstances, the cells lining the breast ducts and lobes multiply only under strictly regulated conditions and in response to specific signals.*

- *Overgrowth of cells may occur in any part of the lobes or ducts, and may progress through four stages.*

- *One: Hyperplasia The cells multiply more than necessary, creating a harmless excess that builds up inside the duct.*

- *Two: Atypical hyperplasia The cells lose their normal appearance and are called "atypical". This is still a benign condition.*

- *Three: Carcinoma in situ The atypical cells fill up the duct, forming a carcinoma, but the cells are not invasive.*

- *Four: Invasive carcinoma The atypical cells break out of the duct and spread to the surrounding tissues. This is a true invasive cancer.*

with mastectomy at a later date, if necessary. Ultimately, the choice of treatment depends on a woman's individual risk, whether she has a family history of breast cancer, whether there is calcification in her breast lesion (see p. 21), and her age when it is found.

Lobular carcinoma in situ (LCIS) LCIS in itself does not develop into cancer, but it is useful as a marker, showing that a woman is at risk of developing DCIS. This explains why breast cancer in women who have been diagnosed with LCIS doesn't always develop in the same spot as the LCIS, or even in the same breast. Because of this, removing the affected lobe will not reduce the risk, so the woman with LCIS is in the same position as other women at high risk. She must either have both breasts removed or have close follow-up, with regular breast self-examination, medical checks and mammograms. Most women opt for the latter.

Ductal carcinoma in situ (DCIS) DCIS represents the far end of the spectrum of hyperplasia (see p. 53); a woman with DCIS has 11 times the normal risk of developing invasive cancer. It is most common in breast ducts adjacent to an established cancer (it is often found when a cancerous lump is removed), and so is nearly always treated by some form of breast surgery. DCIS tends to fall into two distinct types: focal (occurring in only one spot in the breast) and multicentric (in several parts of the breast). There is little tendency for the first to proceed to the second.

Total mastectomy will be recommended for multicentric DCIS. If mammograms do not show clearly which type is present, however, a wide excision of the lump, plus a margin of healthy tissue, will be performed; alternatively, the whole quadrant of the affected breast will be removed. The tissue that has been removed is microscopically examined and, if the DCIS is found to have more than one focus, total mastectomy will be done after discussion with the patient.

If the original area of DCIS is the only focus in all the breast tissue removed, a further surgical procedure may not be recommended. Follow-up is crucial, however, because of the increased risk of invasive cancer. It should take the form of monthly self-examination, yearly clinical examination by a doctor and two-yearly mammography. It is unclear if any additional treatment, such as radiotherapy or tamoxifen, is needed, although one US trial suggests that radiotherapy can reduce local recurrence rates. This topic is the subject of a UK trial; your doctor may ask you to take part in it.

TRUE CANCER

As a rule, breast cancers arise from the cells that line the ducts or lobules. The most frequent form is known as ductal carcinoma because it was originally thought to arise from the milk ducts. It is now recognized, however, that both this type and the less common lobular carcinoma usually arise in the breast lobule. All other forms of breast cancer are rare. Both ductal and lobular carcinomas can be pre-invasive (see LCIS and DCIS, left) or invasive.

Invasive ductal carcinoma   Ductal carcinomas comprise over 80 percent of all detected breast cancers. The first symptom is generally a new, hard, ill-defined lump within the breast. As the tumour spreads along the strands of connective tissue between the breast lobes, it pulls on the overlying skin, creating a characteristic dimpling effect. Extreme skin pitting, known as *peau d'orange* because the skin resembles orange peel, is a serious sign. If the tumour spreads along the ducts, it will pull on and eventually invert the nipple; this is why a new inversion of the nipple should always prompt you to visit your doctor, although it can also be caused by duct ectasia (see p. 36), a benign condition. The lymph nodes under the armpits may be involved, and as the tumour spreads it may also involve the underlying muscles. The smaller and less advanced the cancer is at the time of diagnosis, the better the outlook (see pp. 60–61).

Invasive lobular carcinoma   Lobular carcinomas account for about 10 percent of breast cancers and behave in a very similar way to ductal cancers, except that they may spread diffusely rather than forming a discrete tumour.

SITES OF CANCER

Breast cancer can arise in the lobes or, more rarely, the milk ducts. If it is non-invasive and remains confined to the lobe or duct, it is termed "carcinoma in situ". Once it spreads to the surrounding tissue, it is a true invasive cancer.

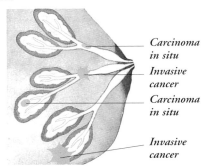

Carcinoma in situ

Invasive cancer

Carcinoma in situ

Invasive cancer

DIAGNOSIS AND BREAST LUMPS

If you report a lump to your doctor, or something shows up on a mammogram, you will be referred to a breast unit. The initial tests that are done depend on whether there is a high probability of cancer.

If cancer is unlikely, fine-needle aspiration cytology (FNAC, see p. 33) is used to take a sample of cells from the lump. Laboratory analysis of the aspirated cells will distinguish between a benign lump and a malignant one.

If cancer is suspected from your mammogram or because of your age or family history, or if FNAC reveals cancer or is inconclusive, a biopsy is needed to provide a sample of tissue from the lump.

A core needle biopsy or open biopsy (see p. 58) is carried out to provide a sample of tissue from the lump. If it can't be felt, wire localization will be used (see column, p. 70).

Following biopsy, histology (analysis of slices of tissue) will diagnose the cancer type and grade the tumour (see p. 60).

Further tests are carried out to see if the cancer has spread (see Diagnosis of secondary spread, p. 59), to determine the outlook for the cancer and to help plan treatment.

DETECTION AND DIAGNOSIS

Mammography is your lifeline. Routine mammographic screening can cut the death rate from breast cancer by 20–30 percent. For example, DCIS (see p. 54) becomes invasive in 50–75 percent of cases within five years, so early detection is crucial. Mammography can detect cancers less than 5 millimetres (¼ inch) across, whereas a lump cannot be felt by either you or your doctor until it has grown to about 1 centimetre (½ inch). In the UK, screening has brought about a marked lowering of the number of women with aggressive tumours and spread to the axilla. Between 30 and 50 percent of detected tumours now measure less than 2 centimetres (¾ inch) when they are first diagnosed; 20 years ago, the proportion was only 5–10 percent.

There are drawbacks to this routine screening, however. Some doctors are concerned about the number of marginal abnormalities detected by mammography, which may then be treated when they should probably be left alone. If surgeons operate on women who have in situ cancers (see p. 54) as if they had invasive breast cancer (perhaps even performing mastectomy), there is the possibility that such women will undergo unnecessary surgery. Despite these questions, you need to remember that mammography is the best screening tool available for the detection of breast cancer and the only screening method for malignancy, the value of which has been proved by rigorous clinical trials.

Special cases for screening Currently, evidence supports the value of two-yearly screening only in women between the ages of 50 and 70, since the incidence of breast cancer is lower in younger women and mammography is less efficient when breast tissue is more dense (as it is in younger women). In some special cases, however, screening should be carried out at an earlier age and more frequently than every three years, which is the recommended interval in the UK.

US guidelines for a woman with a first-degree relative (that is, mother or sister) who develops pre-menopausal breast cancer are that she be routinely screened every two years, starting when she is ten years younger than the age at which her relative developed breast cancer. Women who are diagnosed with atypical hyperplasia (see p. 53) are also advised to have mammography every two years.

Identifying cancer Mammography does not reveal only cancer. It also detects benign lumps, which have rounded, smooth edges and a halo of healthy fat around them. Cancerous lumps, on the other hand, are more dense at the centre than they are at the edges, which are often irregular. Mammography may also be able to show other changes, for instance skin thickening, or tethering and distortion of breast tissue around a lump. A deposit of calcium particles may show up as white dots; this is called calcification. In a benign lump, calcification appears as relatively large blobs; with cancer it has a characteristic fine, speckled appearance. To a radiologist experienced in interpreting mammograms, this almost certainly confirms that the lump is malignant.

DIAGNOSIS

When a woman finds a lump in her breast, doctors use many investigative techniques and skills in order to arrive at as specific a diagnosis as possible. The initial sequence of tests varies, depending on whether the lump has been found by the woman herself or has been detected during routine screening on a mammogram, in which case it may be too small to feel. In all cases, however, a sample of cells or tissue will have to be examined under a microscope to determine whether the lump is malignant; if it is, further tests will be carried out to assess the precise origin of the tumour, its grade and its stage (see pp. 60–61).

Clinical diagnosis The doctor will start his examination by looking at your breasts while you sit with your hands by your sides and then with your arms raised above your head, so that he or she can observe any asymmetry between the breasts, nipple retraction (the nipple will appear drawn in), difference in level between the nipples or dimpling of the skin. If you've been doing regular breast self-examination (see pp. 14–17), you'll be able to confirm which of these features are new and which you have observed in the past.

You will then be asked to lie back with your arms above your head while the doctor examines your breasts carefully, feeling each quadrant of both breasts with the flat of the hand. The aim is to decide whether there is an obvious, discrete lump or if the breasts are just generally lumpy. The doctor will then check the underarm region on both sides for any lumps caused by swollen lymph nodes, the area above the collarbone (this also checks for swollen lymph nodes) and the abdomen and chest (continued p. 58).

BIOFIELD EXAMINATION

Trials are in progress to establish the effectiveness of a new, non-invasive technique to detect breast cancer: breast biofield examination.

Breast biofield examination (BBE) is based on the fact that there is a tiny electric difference between the interior and the exterior of a healthy cell. This is disrupted when the cell becomes cancerous, and the disruption can be detected on the BBE scanner.

In its only full trial, on 392 women with suspicious breast lesions, the scanner had an accuracy rate of 98 percent, pinpointing 178 of the 182 cancers later detected by biopsy.

There are hopes that further successes will mean that BBE will be used more widely in the next year or two. It could be a particularly useful technique for detecting breast cancer in younger women: since their breasts are denser than those of older women, mammograms are not very effective.

CORE NEEDLE BIOPSY

FNAC (see p. 33) yields only a tiny sample of cells from breast tissue, so it's impossible to tell whether they originate from an in situ cancer or an invasive cancer. A core needle biopsy provides a core of cells that can be analysed to make this distinction.

● *Under local anaesthetic, a special fine-notched needle with a sheath is inserted into the lump in order to withdraw a fine core of tissue from it.*

● *The sheath is drawn back and some tissue from the lump falls into the notch.*

● *The sheath is closed, trapping a tiny core of tissue from the lump inside the notch, and the needle is withdrawn.*

● *The skin is left virtually intact. Although there may be a little bruising afterwards, there is hardly any discomfort.*

If your symptoms are lumpiness of the breasts or pain or both, but no obvious new discrete lump is found when the doctor examines you, further management will depend on your age. If you are under the age of 40, cancer is unlikely, and you may be asked to return in six weeks. If you still have pain from a lumpy breast, treatment may be advised (see column, p. 29). If you are over 40, a mammogram may be advised to ensure that no hidden cancer is present. If this shows no evidence of malignancy, you can be reassured and offered treatment for your symptoms if necessary. If there is any suspicion of cancerous pattern on the mammogram, FNAC (see p. 33) will be advised and perhaps further tests, depending on the result of the FNAC.

If you have discharge from the nipple, it will be tested to see if it contains blood (this is not always obvious to the naked eye) and the doctor will note whether the discharge comes from a single duct or many. Nipple discharge is usually associated with benign conditions (see pp. 36–37), but in rare cases a bloodless discharge from either single or multiple ducts may require further investigation to rule out cancer. Laboratory tests of the discharge are too inaccurate to rely on, so your doctor will need to perform a biopsy.

If there is an obvious lump that the doctor can feel, the next step is to biopsy it, usually by aspirating the lump (see column, p. 33). The sample of breast tissue will be sent to the laboratory for microscopic examination.

Open biopsy This kind of biopsy is an alternative to a core needle biopsy (see left). As the name implies, the skin is cut open to reveal the lump and remove it with a margin of healthy breast tissue. In practical terms, therefore, open biopsy nearly always means removing the whole lump (lumpectomy, see p. 71), and this procedure will be carried out in hospital under a general anaesthetic. Not every woman over 30 with an obvious lump should have it removed, however. The aim is to diagnose the lump – lumps that are benign are in the main left alone and not removed.

Complications of open biopsy are rare (fewer than one in ten cases) but, as with any surgical procedure, they do occur. The two most likely are a haematoma (bruise) and, less often, infection. A haematoma forms due to blood oozing into the tissue surrounding the site of the biopsy, and may show up as a bruise with a vague lump beneath within a day or two of a biopsy having been done. As with any other bruise, the body simply absorbs the blood and recycles it, and the bruise will disappear after a week or so. Infection, if it occurs, will probably show up within a week of the biopsy as pain and a raised temperature; it is usually successfully treated with a course of antibiotics. Very rarely, a haematoma may become infected and an abscess may form. Antibiotics will be prescribed and the abscess can be surgically drained (see Nipple infections, pp. 37–38).

Analysing the biopsy The biopsy or lump is sent to the pathology laboratory where it is very finely sliced, stained to show up the cells and examined under a microscope; this process is known as histology. If the tissue is found to be cancerous, a very precise diagnosis of cancer, and the type of cancer it is, can be made. The tumour is also graded (see p. 60), providing information about how malignant it is. At some hospitals, specialized tests (see p. 62) may be performed on a slice of tumour tissue to reveal features that help to decide treatment and give the patient an idea of what the future outlook may be.

An open biopsy is performed purely to remove the lump and send it for analysis. If cancer is found, the surgeon will wait to discuss the treatment options with the woman and her family before any further surgery is carried out. In the past, a biopsy was analysed instantly while the woman was still under general anaesthetic. If the lump proved to be cancerous, mastectomy was performed immediately. This was extremely traumatic and is no longer done.

Diagnosis of secondary spread In addition to lymph node involvement (see p. 74), spread of the disease to the rest of the body is checked by a series of simple tests, which are generally performed during the initial assessment. They include chest X-rays to detect secondary tumours in the lungs or involvement of the membranes around them, and a blood test to look for anaemia or abnormalities of the blood cells, which may indicate that the bone marrow has been invaded. Any abnormalities of blood chemistry that might indicate spread to the bones or liver are picked up at the same time. If a woman has no clinical evidence of metastases (secondary tumours) and her blood tests are normal, the chances are that the cancer has not spread. In more advanced cases, specialized tests are used to check for secondaries, including X-rays or bone scans of likely sites of bone spread (the skull, spine, pelvis and hips) and an ultrasound examination to assess the state of the liver.

ONE-STOP DIAGNOSIS

The world's leading breast units, including the Royal Marsden NHS Trust in London and the Sloan-Kettering Institute in New York, are working towards a 24-hour, one-stop diagnosis for all breast lumps.

A woman referred to the unit with a lump will be given a diagnostic mammogram or ultrasound scan depending on her age, FNAC (see p. 33) and, if this is positive or inconclusive, a core needle biopsy (see column, left).

The material for analysis is sent straight to the laboratory, and a firm diagnosis can be made within 24 hours.

As well as helping doctors, this service reduces the considerable anxiety of waiting for test results to a minimum.

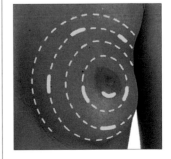

Biopsy incisions
When a biopsy is carried out, the cut is usually made along natural tension lines in the skin of the breast, to help keep scarring to a minimum.

The size of the tumour, the involvement of axillary lymph nodes and the presence of secondary tumours are vital factors in assessing how far the disease has progressed and determining the outlook.

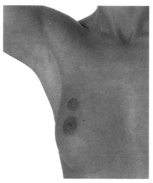

Stage I
The disease is confined to the breast. Dimpling of the skin may or may not be present.

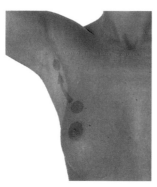

Stage II
The axillary lymph nodes are affected. Stages I and II may be curable by surgery but some adjuvant systemic treatment, such as tamoxifen therapy, is usually advised.

ASSESSMENT

One of the major aims of your doctors will be to get a feel for the "virulence" of your cancer. To do this, they use a series of tests to decide your treatment and assess your long-term outlook. The tests are intended to determine the grade of the tumour, which means the aggressiveness of its cells, and the stage of the disease, which is a measure of how far advanced it is and how far it has spread (if at all) beyond its original site in the breast.

GRADING

When cancer cells are microscopically examined, they can be graded according to their appearance or type. How they look indicates how malignant the cancer is. Generally, the more primitive the cells, the more malignant the cancer.

The degree of cell specialization is known as the grade of the tumour and can give a fairly reliable guide to the long-term outlook for the patient. Tumours of recognizable cells, which look quite similar to their normal cells of origin (that is, breast tissue), are called "well-differentiated" or Grade 1 and carry an excellent outlook. Tumours containing cells that become increasingly unrecognizable as breast tissue are known as "poorly differentiated" or "undifferentiated" and descend through Grades 2 and 3 with a worsening prognosis.

STAGING

Once a breast cancer has been diagnosed and graded, the patient as a whole is staged (see columns left and right). In order to stage every patient individually, three factors are taken into account: the size of the tumour; whether the axillary lymph nodes are involved; and whether there are metastases (secondary tumours) elsewhere in the body.

Although size is a fairly crude predictor of the invasive potential of the tumour, generally speaking the larger the tumour, the more likely it is to have had time to spread to the axillary lymph nodes. Even a small tumour may have spread, however. Most women whose tumours measure less than 1 centimetre (½ inch) and whose axillary lymph nodes are free of disease have an excellent prognosis.

In assessing a patient's outlook, the crucial factor against which all others should be weighed is spread to the axillary lymph nodes; the more nodes that are involved, the worse the prognosis. With a node-negative cancer, seven women out of ten will be alive ten years later; with a node-positive cancer, only five or fewer out of ten. Adjuvant chemotherapy (see pp. 80–81) is now routinely given to pre-menopausal women with involved nodes. Most other women, whether their nodes are free of cancer or not, would benefit from adjuvant systemic therapy, usually tamoxifen (see p. 79).

The presence of metastases elsewhere in the body can be detected by tests (see Diagnosis of secondary spread, p. 59). If the lymph nodes above the collarbone are involved, these are regarded as metastases. Distant metastases in the lungs, liver or bones automatically put the cancer at Stage IV, so their presence is a very serious sign.

Planning treatment Once you have been staged, decisions about treatment can be made. You have the right to discuss all of the possible alternatives so that you and your family participate in all decisions. You can also be helped to come to terms with the diagnosis by being given a tape-recording of the "bad news consultation" to take home, so ask for one, and by having a friend or relative with you for moral support when the news is broken.

Survival Doctors prefer to talk about survival rather than "cure". It is usual to measure five-year and ten-year survival rates and then express them as a percentage. If you are told by your doctor that your cancer has a five-year survival rate of 80 percent, it means this: out of ten women with your disease, with a tumour of the same grade and stage, and of the same degree of aggressiveness, eight could expect to be alive in five years' time.

PROGNOSIS AND OUTLOOK

The stage of the tumour (see right and far left) is crucial in assessing five-year survival rate for breast cancer: the five-year survival rate of 85 percent for women suffering from Stage I tumours falls to less than ten percent for those with Stage IV tumours.

About one in every three women treated vigorously for early breast cancer will go on to have a normal life expectancy. Of the rest, those who get local recurrence can often be treated adequately with radiotherapy. Only about half of the women who see breast-cancer surgeons see them early enough, when the disease is eminently treatable and curable; the other half leave it too long before seeking help (continued p. 62).

ADVANCED STAGES

The stage of the tumour is crucial in assessing five-year survival rate. The prognosis worsens when the disease has invaded the lungs, liver or bones, although breast cancer can defy all predictions.

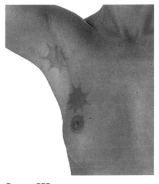

Stage III
The disease has spread and invaded the muscles of the chest wall, the overlying skin, or possibly the lymph nodes above the collarbone.

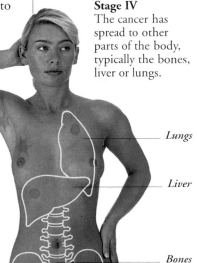

Stage IV
The cancer has spread to other parts of the body, typically the bones, liver or lungs.

Lungs

Liver

Bones

Most women with breast cancer still have a reasonable expectation of life by comparison with cancers of the lung, stomach or ovary. Many women can expect to live in comfort for many years after treatment, even if their disease cannot be classed as cured. Since breast cancer is mainly a disease of older women, many will die from other causes or simply from old age rather than from their breast tumour.

SPECIAL RESEARCH TESTS

Over the years, researchers have attempted to develop special tests that will provide doctors with an even better idea of the aggressiveness of breast tumours, future outlook and survival. The tests require very advanced technology and are by no means performed at all centres, but it is hoped that their future use will help to identify groups of patients who would do better with one kind of treatment or another.

Oestrogen receptors (ERs)　Approximately 60 percent of cancers contain detectable ERs. A tumour that has ERs is sensitive to oestrogen and has a slightly better prognosis than one that doesn't.

Epidermal growth-factor receptor (EGFr)　All cells have receptors that are "switched on" by growth factors telling the cell to multiply. In altered cells, the receptors don't wait for signals, but cause the cells to multiply uncontrollably. About half of all breast-cancer cases have altered receptors. Tumours that are EGFr-negative generally have a better outlook for recovery than those that are positive.

Ki-67　Put simply, this measures the speed of cell growth and division; in general, the faster the cells are dividing, the more aggressive the tumour. The consequence of this is that the spread of the cancer throughout the body is likely to occur earlier and be faster. The chance of metastases is high and the outlook poorer than with slower cell changes.

erbB-2　Research has shown that women who relapse have extra copies of the altered form of this gene, and higher levels of the protein it produces. The more erbB-2 present, the poorer the prognosis seems to be.

Cathepsin D　Patients with low levels of this enzyme and positive axillary nodes invariably outlive those with high levels of cathepsin D and negative nodes. It is therefore quite a powerful predictor of outcome.

p53　This gene mutation is known to be present in about half of all breast cancers. An abnormality of p53 also gives an increased risk of ovarian and bowel cancers.

ON FINDING A LUMP

So much attention is given to breast cancer nowadays in all the popular media that it would be difficult for any woman to ignore the potential significance of a breast lump. The sad fact is that on finding a lump, practically all women underestimate the chances of survival and overestimate the chances of dying. Finding a breast lump is therefore a shocking experience for everyone.

THE IMPLICATIONS OF DELAY

Finding a lump in the breast will always be scary, but don't become so frightened that you don't seek help immediately. It's been estimated that approximately one in five women with symptoms of breast cancer delay seeking advice for three months or more, and some research has suggested that this delay could well be contributing to the high mortality rates from breast cancer in Great Britain.

The interval between finding a breast lump and having a diagnosis confirmed is the most stressful part of finding a lump in your breast. A group of women who were studied before and after having their lump diagnosed as benign were found to suffer severe impairment of critical thinking and concentration, together with profound anxiety before the diagnosis. Fewer than one in eight women gives breast loss as her primary concern; nearly six out of ten are more distressed at the prospect of having cancer.

ON HEARING THE DIAGNOSIS

Individual strategies for coping and personality factors will affect your response to the news that you have breast cancer. Social support can help you, and the communications skills of your medical carers – especially the surgeon who breaks the news – are extremely important. Your reaction may have several stages; denial, fighting back, brave acceptance, depressed acceptance and a mixture of helplessness and hopelessness are all possible.

Most women are likely at some time to go through stages of depressed acceptance, where they acknowledge that they have a potentially fatal disease but are overwhelmed with fears for themselves and their families. At worst, they may feel that there is no hope for them; whatever they have to live for, they may not be able to muster the energy to fight for it by overcoming the disease (continued p. 64).

DENIAL

One of the most common coping strategies is denial, a natural protective mechanism that helps you go on with life in times of stress or shock.

- *You may try to convince yourself that a lump is nothing to worry about until it can no longer be ignored. Such delay in reporting symptoms will worsen the outlook.*

- *By the time you seek help, the tumour is difficult to treat and the chances of survival are therefore much lower.*

- *Individuals most likely to delay reporting a breast lump include older women; women of lower social class or little education; women who are fearful of cancer and surgery and don't feel they can be helped or cured; women who are inhibited about their bodies; depressed or anxious personalities or those who habitually resort to denial when faced with a crisis.*

- *Paradoxically, knowledge as opposed to ignorance about breast cancer may inhibit some women from seeking advice at the proper time; one study showed that female healthcare professionals, especially nurses, tended to report their lumps later and generally had larger tumours than other women.*

SUPPORT

Women who have supportive family and friends are more able to cope with this kind of life crisis. Hearing the bad news in the presence of a close relative or friend reduces anxiety and depression for a long time afterwards, and he or she will probably remember more clearly than you what the doctor said. The presence of a trusted ally, be it spouse, partner, friend or relative, is useful in the long term to help you accept that you have cancer.

THE FAMILY

The needs of your family are sometimes overlooked. It's easy to assume that they will be able to keep their feelings in check and be ready to offer you support. Families do, however, suffer along with you and very often reflect your mood. One study showed that if a patient with cancer is depressed or anxious there is a very high probability that the next of kin will be also.

Partners   Your spouse or partner is likely to feel responsible for helping you to adjust successfully to your disease and to your new body after any necessary surgery. He may suffer considerable emotional distress but pretend to hide this behind a confident pose, assuming that this will help you. Unfortunately this attitude may lead to misunderstandings. You may feel that your partner is not being sensitive to your feelings and doesn't realize the seriousness of the situation or can't share your fears. It is natural when a loved one is in distress to try to offer advice, be cheery, or somehow "sort things out", but this may not be what you need; more often you just want someone to listen and understand.

Close relationships are always affected in some way by a diagnosis of breast cancer; with fragile relationships, this burden may prove to be the final straw. For the majority of women, however, this is a time when the commitment, love and affection of her family and friends are re-affirmed.

At the time the diagnosis is made, good information and counselling should be provided to the person closest to you, since this "significant other" will be a crucial factor in your long-term adjustment. In the end, most couples feel their relationships to be at least the same as before diagnosis, and sometimes even better.

"Waiting for the diagnosis was pure hell. I lay awake at night imagining the cancer was spreading through my body. Nothing could distract me for more than a few minutes – not work, not my family or my friends. I'd been decorating the spare bedroom because my parents were coming to stay, and I just didn't have the heart to go on with it. I kept thinking about what I might have to tell them."

Jill, 36, Potter

TREATING BREAST CANCER

The detection and diagnosis of breast cancer is only the first step in combating the disease. You have the right to expect the best possible care. All women should know what their treatment options are – including a clear and detailed explanation of the aims of the proposed treatments, their benefits and any possible side-effects – and have the opportunity to discuss treatment plans with interested and sympathetic breast-care specialists. They should also know what techniques are involved, the impact of treatment and the support they are entitled to receive, especially when coming to terms with life after treatment.

When you find a lump in your breast, you are entitled to the best possible treatment. Your care should include:

• *A prompt referral by your family doctor to a team specializing in the diagnosis and treatment of breast cancer, including a consultant.*

• *A firm diagnosis within one week of being examined.*

• *The opportunity of a confirmed diagnosis before consenting to any form of treatment, including surgery.*

• *Full information about types of surgery (including breast reconstruction where appropriate) and the role of adjuvant treatments such as radiotherapy, chemotherapy, hormone therapy including tamoxifen, and so on.*

• *A clear and detailed explanation of the aims of the proposed treatments and their benefits and any possible side-effects (including long term).*

TREATMENT OPTIONS

If you are diagnosed as having breast cancer, it's crucial that you are fully aware of the various treatment options that are open to you. Twenty years ago, radical mastectomies were the rule; today, surgery aims to conserve the breast if at all possible. At the same time, very sophisticated reconstructive surgery has been developed so that a woman who loses her breast has the option of replacing it. Advanced techniques for calculating future risks mean that doctors can place a woman in a very clearly defined group and choose a tailor-made treatment programme especially for her, giving her the best possible chance of a cure.

BREAST UNITS

Women with breast cancer are increasingly treated at specialist units, such as those at Guy's Hospital in London and the Sloan-Kettering Institute in New York. These units offer the best possible care and ensure close co-operation between an interested and sympathetic oncologist, surgeon, pathologist, radiologist and radiotherapist, which allows rapid and accurate diagnosis and appropriate treatment. The team will also include special breast-care nurses or counsellors who deal with the emotional and psychological aspects of breast cancer. Specialist breast cancer units also supervise adjuvant therapy (additional forms of treatment) such as radiotherapy, chemotherapy and hormone therapy, and can arrange for breast reconstruction if desired, so that all your treatments are kept under one roof with a minimum of travel and disturbance during follow-up.

CONSERVING THE BREAST

Women who develop breast cancer today are in a much more fortunate position than in the past; many more treatment options are open to you and preserving the breast need pose no hazard to life. Not so long ago it was thought that mastectomy, including the removal of all the axillary lymph nodes, was necessary in every case to give a woman the best chance of survival. This is no longer true. Doctors have abandoned the idea that this kind of extensive surgery should be routine and – without sacrificing results – have greatly improved recovery after surgery. With conservative treatment, the once worst complication of breast surgery, swelling of the arm (see Lymphoedema, p. 88) is now rare.

Surgeons today believe in conserving the breast whenever possible or choosing the least extensive operation that is appropriate. With early breast cancer, lumpectomy is nearly always an option. This means that very small tumours can be dealt with, leaving the breast virtually intact.

Because the many different approaches to treatment all offer about the same success rate, there's nothing to prevent your preferences about the choice of operation from carrying weight. The outlook for the disease is affected more by the grade and stage of the tumour (see pp. 60–61) when it is diagnosed than by the type of surgery performed.

Any choice should be made in consultation with you and with your family. Not all patients are suitable for breast conservation, however, and you would be well advised to listen to your doctors if they advocate a more radical approach. If lumpectomy is attempted in inappropriate cases (on a large tumour, for example), the cosmetic results and control of the disease can be poor.

THE LOSS OF A BREAST

Whenever the subject of mastectomy is discussed, be sure that you and your family understand precisely the extent of the operation. Ask to see some photographs of women after mastectomy, to give you an idea of how your body will look after surgery. You'll almost certainly need time, space and counselling to get used to the idea of a different-looking body, which at first may seem alien to you.

You'll have much greater difficulty coming to terms with your new appearance than your partner, family and friends will. They are far more concerned about your well-being and long-term health than about your body's appearance. It's understandable, however, that you are not. A woman's self-image is often indistinguishable from her self-esteem. Fortunately, doctors and surgeons now understand this and should be willing to give you all the help you need.

You are entitled to have a cosmetically acceptable result after surgery and to be pleased with your appearance when dressed, even in low necklines. This can be achieved with prostheses (see p. 89). Reconstructive surgery (see p. 82) is also widely available to restore both breast contour and a nipple if you so wish. Don't be afraid to ask your surgeon about these things or worry that you will be thought vain or frivolous. You have the right to expect your surgeon to be sympathetic to these concerns, and most surgeons are.

CONSIDERING TREATMENT

Whatever your doctors advise, your have the right to time, space and counselling when considering treatment. Your care should include:

- *Access to a specialist breast-care nurse trained to give you information and emotional and psychological support.*

- *As much time as you need to consider your treatment options and gather information.*

- *A sensitive and complete breast prosthesis service, where appropriate.*

- *The opportunity to meet a former breast-cancer patient who has been trained to offer practical, psychological and emotional support.*

- *Information on all support services (including local and national groups) available to breast-cancer patients and their families.*

BREAST CANCER IN PREGNANCY

It seems that breast cancer is no more likely to arise in pregnancy and behaves no differently during pregnancy than at any other time. Be assured that the hormonal changes of pregnancy, when levels of oestrogen are high, do not seem to make the situation worse.

There is no good reason why breast cancer in pregnant women should routinely lead to termination.

The toxic anti-cancer drugs used in chemotherapy do affect the developing fetus and it therefore seems best to avoid this kind of medication in the first three months of pregnancy. After three months, selected and well-tried drugs may be given with safety.

Generally, radiotherapy is not considered an option in the first six months of pregnancy; even in the last three months, its use is controversial.

An alternative approach would be to perform a mastectomy rather than just a lumpectomy, since this would avoid the need for radiotherapy to the breast (see p. 78).

CONSIDERING CANCER TREATMENT

When your doctors consider the treatment of your breast cancer, they are taking into consideration several different factors that will influence the treatment you have and your long-term outlook. Doctors have to tread a narrow line between establishing the most effective treatment for your condition and needing to cause you the least trauma, both physical and mental. This fine balance is not always easy to achieve and requires your full and frank input as well as your co-operation. In addition, the better informed you are about the issues involved, the more active a part you can take in deciding your own treatment. This will not only help your doctor and surgeon in their task but may also give you added strength in fighting and overcoming your cancer. The first thing you need to understand is that treatment of breast cancer falls into three distinct areas:

• treatment of the lump, usually with surgery
• treatment of the lymph nodes in the axilla if they are involved in the cancer, with surgical clearance as a rule
• adjuvant (additional) therapy where appropriate, which could be radiotherapy to clear any remaining cancer cells from the breast after surgery, or chemotherapy or hormone therapy (with a drug such as tamoxifen) to catch any spread of the cancer to the rest of the body.

Surgery and radiotherapy are both referred to as local treatments, since they treat only the area where the tumour has occurred. Chemotherapy and hormone therapy are both called systemic treatments, since they treat the whole of the body, not just the diseased part.

The state-of-the-art treatment for breast cancer appears to be the one pioneered by Guy's Hospital in London and centres in Paris, Milan, and Boston in the US. The first step is exact diagnosis with cutting-needle biopsy (see p. 58), done under local anaesthetic; a short while later (three to seven days), after you have been fully consulted, a single operation under general anaesthetic will remove the lump and clear the axillary lymph nodes. Precise radiotherapy to the tumour site is given, which avoids excessive irradiation of the skin and deeper organs. This gives results at least as good as mastectomy and with much less heartache. Nearly every woman is considered for some form of systemic adjuvant treatment (see p. 77–81). If you have a tumour less than 1 centimetre (½ inch) in diameter and are node-negative (that is, the cancer has not spread to the axillary lymph nodes), you belong to the only group of women for whom systemic therapy is not considered necessary.

PLANNING TREATMENT

Breast cancer is usually referred to as early or advanced; this reflects whether the tumour is operable or not. "Early" usually encompasses Stages I and II and "advanced", Stages III and IV (see pp. 60–61). These terms are also used to reflect the aggressiveness of the tumour – some patients do quite well with large, ulcerated cancers that have been present for some time but which are clearly not rapidly growing because they have not spread. A small primary tumour, on the other hand, can spread quickly to other organs if it is very aggressive. With early breast cancer (see right), local control is of prime importance and, as proven at Guy's Hospital, can be achieved largely by removal of the lump with a margin of healthy breast tissue, followed by a course of radiotherapy in some form. If you have a large or aggressive tumour, you'll be asked to consider mastectomy. All patients except those with very early cancer will be given adjuvant therapy in some form; for nearly all older women, this is the drug tamoxifen (see pp. 79–80).

If a tumour is allowed to reach an advanced state, then the likelihood of metastases (secondary tumours) is much greater. For this reason, local treatment alone is deemed inadequate and systemic treatment is the rule. The most common systemic treatment for pre-menopausal women is chemotherapy. This works on cancer throughout the whole body and may shrink your tumour to an operable size.

PRIMARY MEDICAL THERAPY

Research at the excellent breast unit in Milan, Italy, showed that chemotherapy given *before* the operation can reduce four out of five large tumours to less than 3 centimetres (1½ inches) in diameter, allowing them to be treated with more conservative surgery and therefore reducing physical and emotional trauma. Tumours have been clearly seen to shrink and disappear on successive mammograms, although microcalcification (see p. 21) may remain. Primary medical treatment, where practised, is always followed by additional surgical treatment to avoid the chance of local relapse.

TREATING EARLY BREAST CANCER

The treatment of early breast cancer – that is, a cancer that has not yet spread beyond the axillary lymph nodes – has three main aims:

- *to control the disease locally (this means at the site of the tumour) and prevent local recurrence.*

- *to treat any micrometastatic disease (tiny, undetectable secondary spread) so as to increase the chances of survival.*

- *to conserve as much of the breast as possible and be minimally disfiguring.*

IMPALPABLE LESIONS

Lesions that can't be felt by physical examination, but show up on mammography as shadows with tiny white dots of calcification, can be accurately located with mammographic guidance.

• *Small solid tumours can also be localized with the use of ultrasound and a small wire (see photograph below).*

• *The surgeon dissects down onto the wire so that the whole of the tumour can be cut out, and removes 1–2 centimetres (½–1 inch) of tissue around it. This is then X-rayed while the patient is still anaesthetized to confirm that the abnormality has been completely removed. With this technique, complete excision (removal) in almost 100 percent of impalpable cancers can be achieved.*

Locating the lesion

Using an ultrasound image for guidance, the radiologist inserts a fine wire into the centre of the tumour. The wire is left in place to guide the surgeon to the tumour.

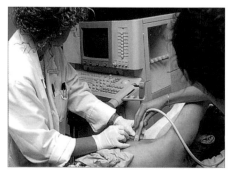

SURGERY

In most cases, local conservative therapy is achieved with surgery. Although it is possible to treat even small tumours with chemotherapy and radiotherapy, these treatments are time-consuming and tend to be reserved for tumours that are greater than 4 centimetres (2 inches) in diameter. In addition, large doses of radiotherapy can produce distortion and disfigurement of the breast tissue.

Lumpectomy is the most common primary treatment for smaller breast cancers and can generally be relied on to give a good cosmetic result (see right). If yours is a large tumour in the centre of the breast or one with several different areas of focus, a mastectomy may be better. A lumpectomy in such instances may not be cosmetically attractive and it may be impossible to provide a satisfactory prosthesis for a very distorted breast. Reconstruction is always an option either during the initial surgery or later. Chemotherapy or hormone therapy prior to surgery may be offered if you have a large tumour, to reduce its size and allow a smaller area of breast tissue to be removed.

Mastectomy is major surgery and you deserve to have an expert, rather than general, surgeon. A British study in 1995 recommended that women with breast cancer be treated only by doctors who see more than 30 new cancers a year, who can offer a full range of treatment options and who work within a team of specialists.

CONSERVATIVE THERAPY

Breast conservation is most suitable if your lump is less than 4 centimetres (2 inches) in diameter, felt on clinical examination or shown on a mammogram. Minimal nodal involvement with no distant metastases (to the liver, lungs or bones) is a requirement. If you have large breasts and a tumour greater than 4 centimetres (2 inches), you might also be suitable. There is no age limit. If you are elderly, provided you are fit, you should be treated in exactly the same way as younger patients.

Breast conservation will not be offered if it would result in an unacceptable cosmetic result. This would normally include the majority of cancers in the centre of the breast and those that are over 4 centimetres (2 inches) in diameter.

Women with more than one focus of cancer have a high local recurrence rate with breast conservation and are better treated with mastectomy, ideally with immediate breast reconstruction (this means during the initial surgery rather than at a later date). Cancer in both breasts can be treated by a bilateral conservation, but you may prefer bilateral mastectomy, again with immediate reconstruction.

LUMPECTOMY

Wherever possible, lumpectomy is now the treatment of choice for breast cancer, because of its cosmetic qualities and because it is less emotionally traumatic. As long as the post-operative dose of radiotherapy is sufficiently high, only the lump itself need be removed, but most surgeons still go for the safety margin of 1 centimetre (½ inch) of normal breast tissue around it. The minimum amount of skin is removed to give the best cosmetic result.

When a large amount of skin needs to be removed (if the lump is very near the surface, for example), the cosmetic results are likely to be rather poor and your doctor should make you aware of this. Most surgeons remove the lymph nodes from the armpit at the same time. The operation itself is a fairly minor procedure carried out under general anaesthetic, and you'll probably have to stay in hospital for four or five days to make sure the scar is healing and there are no complications.

MASTECTOMY

In the past, mastectomy was the treatment of choice for breast cancer, since it was thought that the tumour spread by growing outwards from the primary growth in the centre. It therefore seemed logical to perform ever more extensive surgery in an attempt to get beyond the growing edge of the tumour. Radical surgery is no longer the norm for breast cancer and there are currently several possible variations of mastectomy.

• A partial mastectomy (see also p. 72), as its name implies, involves removing part of the breast (other versions of this type of operation remove varying amounts of tissue). A sample of the axillary nodes will be taken at the same time or the nodes may be cleared. The operation can leave a misshapen breast, depending on how much tissue is removed. Knowing this, women frequently opt for a total mastectomy (continued p. 72).

BREAST SURGERY

There are several possible operations but in all cases, surgeons will aim to remove the minimum amount of tissue that is necessary to get rid of the cancer. The extent of the surgery is determined by the size and position of the tumour, whether the lump has a well-defined outline, how aggressive it appears to be and whether the cancer has spread.

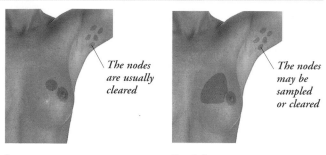

The nodes are usually cleared

The nodes may be sampled or cleared

Lumpectomy
The lump is removed with a 1 centimetre (½ inch) margin of healthy tissue to give the best cosmetic result. The axillary nodes are usually cleared too.

Partial mastectomy
Where the cancer doesn't have a well-defined outline, the lump is removed with a larger amount of surrounding tissue than for a lumpectomy. The axillary nodes are also sampled (see p. 74) or cleared.

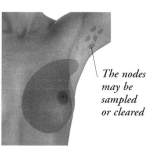

The nodes may be sampled or cleared

Simple or total mastectomy
All of the breast tissue is removed, including the nipple and areola and the axillary tail; the pectoralis minor muscle is not removed. The axillary lymph nodes may be sampled or cleared.

Pectoralis minor muscle removed from behind breast and pectoralis major muscle

The nodes are cleared

Modified radical mastectomy
All of the breast tissue is removed (as with simple mastectomy) and the pectoralis minor muscle. The axillary lymph nodes are cleared.

• A simple or total mastectomy (see above) removes all of the breast tissue including the nipple and areola and the axillary tail. Some or all of the axillary lymph nodes will be cleared (removed) at the same time.
• A modified radical mastectomy (see above) is a total mastectomy. In addition, the pectoralis minor muscle is removed to facilitate complete axillary clearance (removal). This is the favoured operation of many breast units where lumpectomy is not feasible.

• In a radical mastectomy, the pectoralis major muscle is also removed. This extensive operation should probably never be carried out nowadays, however, so don't agree to it without first asking for a second opinion.

Mastectomy is a major operation and you'll have to stay in hospital for four to eight days depending on the type of surgery performed. If your shoulder is stiff afterwards you can do exercises to get it back to normal (see p. 90).

TIMING THE OPERATION

The team at Guy's Hospital, London, first came up with research findings suggesting that pre-menopausal women who had breast surgery during the second half of the menstrual cycle – the so-called luteal phase – had improved survival rates. Their initial findings have now been corroborated by teams in Milan, and at the Sloan-Kettering Institute in New York. The crucial factor seems to be the higher progesterone levels that occur in the luteal phase, and these are linked to a significantly better life expectancy in women with lymph nodes affected by cancer (see p. 74).

A WORD ABOUT MASTECTOMY

More than 80 percent of breast cancers are localized and caught early enough to be suitable for lumpectomy, yet the American College of Surgeons says that only 35 percent are treated in this way. In New York, hospitals just miles apart have widely varying rates for lumpectomy. Why? In Colorado, where three-quarters of women have mastectomies, studies show that it is doctors who are responsible for such low lumpectomy rates, advocating mastectomies even though the profession has had scientific evidence since 1989 to show that lumpectomy plus radiation is just as good as mastectomy. According to some professors in the US, this is because surgeons have not been keeping up to date with medical literature. This is sad because a study has revealed that, when asked, half of mastectomy patients said they'd choose lumpectomy if they could make the decision again.

In 1992, a report in the *New England Journal of Medicine* showed that teaching hospitals, where surgeons tend to keep more up to date, have a higher lumpectomy rate. And women who have lumpectomies return to everyday life more quickly and report better sex lives. You always have the right to a lumpectomy if you're eligible, but you may

TREATING THE AXILLA

A lymph node infiltrated by cancer has ceased to perform any useful service to your body. Furthermore, cancer can only spread further. Affected axillary lymph nodes must therefore be removed or treated vigorously. The treatment of axillary lymph nodes is still debated by surgeons and radiotherapists. The surgical options range from sampling, that is, the removal of a limited number of nodes (with or without subsequent radiotherapy) to complete surgical clearance of the axillary nodes. Some radiotherapists would advocate radiotherapy as the first and only treatment. The consensus among specialists in the UK, however, is that complete axillary node clearance should be the first step in treating the axilla, wherever possible.

All doctors treating breast cancer are concerned to know the status of the axillary nodes because it remains the single best predictor of long-term survival. Added to this, some of the most important treatment choices and decisions are based on axillary node status. In order to get a true idea of the axillary node status, some form of surgical sampling is needed, since as yet there are no good imaging techniques for the axilla. The role of axillary surgery is therefore twofold: to stage the tumour and to treat axillary disease. Radiotherapy may treat the axilla effectively enough, but it precludes staging of the tumour – information that most oncologists consider crucial.

STAGING THE AXILLA

The most accurate way to stage the axilla is to examine the lymph nodes, starting with the shallowest – Level I – and working through to progressively deeper levels; III is the deepest. On average, there are 14 lymph nodes at Level I, five at Level II, and two at Level III. When lymph nodes at Level I are not affected by cancer, the chance of disease at Levels II and III is very slight. However, when five nodes are positive at Level I, there is an 85 percent chance of positive nodes at Levels II and III.

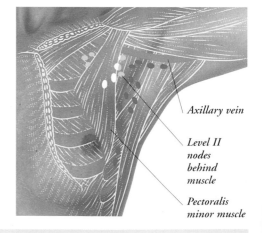

Axillary vein

Level II nodes behind muscle

Pectoralis minor muscle

KEY			
LEVEL I	LEVEL II	LEVEL III	

Logically, then, surgery is superior to radiotherapy, and many surgeons feel that if they are going to operate on the axilla, complete clearance of the lymph nodes gives a better outlook and chance of survival than just sampling.

DETERMINING SPREAD

Sampling of lymph nodes at Level I (see left) can be a good indication of how far the tumour has spread. Surgical options include single-node biopsy, removing a sample of four nodes, Level I clearance, Level II clearance and Level III clearance. Where surgery is the preferred treatment to radiotherapy, then it's obvious that complete clearance rather than sampling is necessary.

Even a single positive lymph node at Level I may be an indication of involvement at Levels II and III. To be sure that there is no involvement at the deeper levels, however, a large sample of clear nodes is required. Research from Edinburgh, Scotland and Denmark has shown that at least ten lymph nodes at Level I have to be sampled in order to give 90 percent confidence in predicting that there is no lymphatic spread of the breast tumour.

There is a direct relationship between the size of your tumour and whether it has already spread to the axillary lymph nodes. If your tumour was detected by screening, however, it's less likely to have axillary spread than if you'd found it yourself, regardless of its size. For this reason, it has become standard practice in many breast units for patients with breast cancer that cannot be felt to have an axillary node sample taken at Level I as a first step. Patients with obvious lumps are treated with Level III clearance.

TREATMENT OF AXILLARY DISEASE

If disease is found in the axillary lymph nodes, there are two main options for treatment: radical radiotherapy and full Level III axillary clearance. Both give good results, but studies have shown that complete axillary clearance gives lower recurrence rates. It provides more information about ultimate outlook and the need for adjuvant therapy, and it avoids the skin irritation and scarring of radiotherapy. The differences, however, are not dramatic and a 95 percent control rate up to ten years is possible using radiotherapy.

Although surgeons may feel zealous about clearing every scrap of cancerous tissue from a woman's body, there is no doubt that those women who have radiotherapy *and*

RECURRENCE IN THE AXILLA

Do discuss how your doctors intend to treat your axilla so that you are aware of what the treatments mean.

- *With no cancer in the lymph nodes, there is only a small difference in rates of recurrence between surgical clearance and radiotherapy.*

- *With involved nodes, surgical clearance will give you a lower chance of recurrence than radiotherapy.*

- *Bear in mind how mobile you want to be and ask about post-treatment complications.*

- *Also consider whether or not you would like to have breast reconstruction (see pp. 82–85).*

axillary surgery suffer as a result. Complications from the treatment include swelling of the arm (see Lymphoedema, p. 88), damage to the nerves in the axilla and a reduction in the range of movement in the shoulder. The aim of treating the axilla must therefore be to control disease with the minimum number of post-operative complications.

SURGERY

If you appear to be node-negative, then it's best that your status is determined by the most limited surgery possible, that is, an axillary lymph-node sample. A Level I sample alone can never be considered a safe procedure in a woman who has a single positive axillary node, because the positive node may imply the presence of disease at Levels II and III. This is why complete surgical clearance is preferred to both stage and treat the axilla.

If you're having a lumpectomy, partial mastectomy or total mastectomy for invasive breast cancer, you should have an axillary clearance, thus avoiding the need for radiotherapy after surgery. This is particularly important when you've opted for immediate breast reconstruction (see p. 82), since radiotherapy will significantly affect the cosmetic result.

It may seem like a contradiction that doctors remove the lymph nodes when their purpose is to fight disease, but in medical terms it makes sense. If they have been infiltrated by cancer, they are no longer useful in any case.

THE PLACE OF RADIOTHERAPY

The medical world is somewhat divided as to whether the axilla should be treated surgically or with radiotherapy. If radiotherapy is done without surgery having determined whether the cancer has spread to the axilla, there is a danger that women without axillary disease will be unnecessarily exposed to radiation and any side-effects; four out of ten women do not have axillary spread.

A sensible approach to treatment, therefore, would be radical radiotherapy to the axilla where surgery determines cancer spread, and a "watch policy" for women who are node-negative. Treatment can thus be limited to patients who have axillary disease or develop it later. The watch policy has been justified by clinical trials that showed no difference in overall survival at ten years between women having radiotherapy initially and women who were given radiotherapy only when monitoring revealed cancer spread.

ADJUVANT THERAPY

Most women with breast cancer will have some form of surgery to remove the tumour, either by taking out the lump alone or by removing the whole breast. By the time the breast cancer is diagnosed, however, some of the cells may have spread beyond the lump itself so there is a risk that some cancer cells may be left behind after surgery.

In about 40 percent of cases where a cancer appears to involve only a single site within one breast, there may be other areas of change in the same breast that are either pre-malignant or already cancerous. Doctors know that, even when the spread of the tumour is not detectable, in many cases cancer has already spread to distant parts of the body, since secondaries appear later on. It may be that, by the time a cancer can be felt, in up to 70 percent of cases small deposits of cancer cells have spread through the body by way of the bloodstream and lymphatic system.

If these cells are allowed to grow, cancer could come back at the same site (local recurrence) or could spread to form secondary tumours (metastases) elsewhere in the body. For this reason, additional forms of treatment are often given as an insurance policy to destroy any remaining cancer cells, wherever they are. This is called *adjuvant* treatment, and it has three main forms:
- radiotherapy given to the breast area to reduce the risk of local recurrence
- hormone treatment
- chemotherapy (cytotoxic drugs).

Hormone treatment and chemotherapy are both *systemic* treatments, aimed at reducing the risk of secondary growth elsewhere in the body. Some form of systemic treatment is probably advisable for most patients, even after surgery and radiotherapy combined, because they can reduce the odds of dying in any year by 25 percent. After ten years, one in ten deaths could be avoided. In the UK, 2,000 lives every year could be saved by using systemic adjuvant therapy.

Ideally, an anti-cancer therapy should be able to kill off only cells affected by the disease without harming healthy cells in the body. Unfortunately no anti-cancer treatment is that discriminating, so some healthy cells are bound to be affected, sometimes leading to side-effects (see Side-effects of chemotherapy, p. 81). Discuss these with your doctor before deciding to proceed with any treatment.

A BOOSTER DOSE OF RADIATION

When a lumpectomy is performed, your surgeon is faced with the dilemma of trying to take as little healthy tissue as is possible to retain the shape of the breast, yet removing enough tissue to ensure maximum safety.

• *Some surgeons feel they can strike the optimum compromise if a booster dose of radiation is given to completely smash any remaining cancer cells.*

• *The booster dose is given in addition to the standard course of radiotherapy.*

• *The boost can be given in several ways, but common to all methods is the delivery of a large dose of extra radiation in a short time.*

• *In Europe, 60 percent of centres use electron therapy. It is very precise and leaves the lungs unharmed (radiation can scar tissue at the top of the lungs).*

• *Other centres have tried implanting tubes at the site of surgery, which can be loaded with radioactive material after the operation. This procedure has proved to be very labour-intensive, involving specially designated treatment areas, and is therefore not practised widely.*

RADIOTHERAPY

Adjuvant radiotherapy is given to catch any cancer cells that may have been left behind after surgery. Doctors now know that simple mastectomy plus local radiotherapy is just as effective a treatment as radical mastectomy, both in terms of controlling local spread and survival rates. A UK study involving nearly 3,000 women showed that there was no difference in survival rates between the two treatments, but showed a marked improvement in controlling local recurrence in women who received radiotherapy.

At one time, radiotherapy was standard treatment after all mastectomies, but now doctors are more selective. If you fulfil any of the following criteria, you'll be a candidate for post-operative radiotherapy:
• a tumour more than 4 centimetres (2 inches) in diameter
• a Grade 3 tumour (see p. 60)
• a node-positive tumour, especially if the disease has spread beyond the axillary lymph nodes.
Even so, deciding who is to be given radiotherapy is not a cut-and-dried procedure, because only about one-third of women with breast cancer are at risk of recurrence. This means that many women would receive unnecessary doses of radiation if all patients were treated.

There's no doubt that radiotherapy should be given to high-risk women with aggressive tumours. For women at lower risk – those with a small, node-negative tumour, for example – it's probably safe to monitor them closely and use radiotherapy only if the cancer returns. Although your hopes may be dashed by local recurrence, try not to get too depressed. It doesn't seem to affect long-term survival rates, provided you get radiotherapy at the time of recurrence.

HOW RADIOTHERAPY IS GIVEN

The aim of adjuvant radiation treatment is to ensure that all the cancer cells in the area of the affected breast are destroyed. Doses of high-energy X-rays are accurately beamed at the breast area of the chest wall and occasionally the axilla and the area above the collarbone. An average course of radiotherapy involves five out-patient treatments each week over about six weeks. Each dose of radiation is meticulously calculated and is then precisely delivered to the area of your skin, which will have been marked with a tiny tattoo of blue dye. Each session can take several minutes, depending on your individual treatment, during which time you will have to lie very still. Otherwise, the experience is not different from that of having an ordinary X-ray. You will be asked not to wash the area during the treatment to avoid irritating the skin. Radiation treatment will not make you radioactive, and there is no danger to adults or children from coming into contact with you.

SYSTEMIC ADJUVANT TREATMENT

The word systemic means affecting the whole. Systemic adjuvant treatment aims to kill off cancer cells throughout your body, thereby preventing any cells that have migrated from the original tumour from causing secondary tumours (metastases) in the bones and organs such as the lungs or liver. The type of systemic treatment that you're eligible for is largely determined by your age. If you are under 50 and pre-menopausal, chemotherapy has been shown to have the most dramatic effect in reducing your odds of dying from the cancer. If you are post-menopausal, hormone treatment in the form of tamoxifen has the same life-saving effect when used for at least two years, especially in tumours that are hormone-sensitive.

HORMONE TREATMENT

Breast cancers may sometimes be influenced by the levels and fluctuations of a woman's hormones, and so lowering oestrogen levels in a woman's body may help in combatting some forms of breast cancer. A few breast cancers are very sensitive to oestrogen levels, and various forms of treatment are aimed at reducing or abolishing a woman's oestrogen production. These include:
- anti-oestrogen drugs such as tamoxifen (the first option)
- surgical removal of the ovaries
- destruction of the ovaries by radiotherapy
- treatment with drugs to stop oestrogen production.

Tamoxifen This drug blocks the stimulatory effect of oestrogen on breast-cancer cells, and it may also have other actions – stimulating the body's own anti-cancer defences, for example. During the last twelve years, tamoxifen has produced a modest but extremely exciting breakthrough in breast-cancer treatment. A single 20-milligram tablet taken daily for between two and five years offers a 20–30 percent reduction in the risk of dying from breast cancer. This appears to continue for at least ten years (continued p. 80).

SIDE-EFFECTS OF RADIATION

Radiotherapy to the breast area does not cause infertility, nor will your hair fall out. You could find the treatments very tiring, so it's a good idea to put aside rest time on your return from hospital and to be relaxed about chores.

- *Occasionally, sickness or nausea follows treatment and meals have to be planned carefully around each session. Anti-nausea tablets will help.*

- *Skin exposed to radiotherapy may become darker, slightly itchy and sore, as though it had been sunburned. Women with fair skin, particularly those with red hair, are more likely to have skin problems than darker-skinned women.*

- *Small blood vessels in the skin may dilate and burst, forming tiny red marks.*

- *The top of the lungs can be affected because radiation can cause scarring while treatment is in progress, leaving behind a dry cough or breathlessness. This may take a few months to clear up.*

- *Radiotherapy has the potential to interfere with the body's immune system, but this side-effect is now very rare.*

- *Any side-effects will usually subside within a few weeks of your stopping radiotherapy, and by no means everyone experiences them.*

- *After finishing radiotherapy, don't expose the treated skin to the sun for about 18 months.*

Tamoxifen produces few side-effects, although some pre-menopausal women may experience menopausal symptoms such as irregular periods and hot flushes. It acts similarly to natural oestrogen and thus reduces the risk of heart disease and prevents post-menopausal bone loss (osteoporosis).

The benefits of tamoxifen apply to all women regardless of age or the stage of their cancer, but women over the age of 50 seem to gain most. The majority of post-menopausal women are therefore given tamoxifen for at least two years after breast-cancer surgery, irrespective of tumour grade, stage or lymph-node involvement. The role of tamoxifen in pre-menopausal women is less certain. However, tamoxifen is now being studied as a way of preventing breast cancer in high-risk groups (see p. 51).

Destruction of the ovaries (ablation) Abolishing the secretion of oestrogen by the ovaries with either surgery or radiotherapy has been shown to increase the overall survival rate for pre-menopausal women with breast cancer by about 10 percent. It also reduces the number of women who get a recurrence by about 25 percent. Most specialists prefer not to use this treatment in younger women unless they are at very high risk because it causes an immediate menopause and loss of fertility.

Goserelin Injecting the drug, goserelin, inhibits the brain hormones that control the ovaries' production of oestrogen. The reduction in oestrogen levels may cause menopausal symptoms in pre-menopausal women. However, the effects are reversible when treatment is stopped. Treatment will continue depending on its efficacy and side-effects.

CHEMOTHERAPY

This treatment, mainly for younger women, uses cytotoxic drugs that find and kill cancer cells anywhere in the body. They are often given after breast-cancer surgery, especially to pre-menopausal women whose axillary lymph nodes are involved or who have particularly aggressive tumours. Chemotherapy will delay relapse by 30 percent and lower the risk of dying by up to 25 percent.

If you do not want surgery or your tumour is unsuitable for surgery, chemotherapy may be the first or only treatment. Since there are many anti-cancer drugs, which are used in different combinations, success rates and side-effects vary. Prolonged multiple drug treatment (cyclical combination chemotherapy), with a combination of cyclophosphamide, methotrexate and 5-fluorouracil (known as CMF), is the most commonly used regimen. The drugs used should be discussed in some detail with your doctor and all possible side-effects carefully considered.

Treatment Adjuvant chemotherapy is usually given by injection or through a drip inserted into a vein in your arm. Treatment tends to be given in cycles at monthly intervals for six months. Although out-patient treatment is possible, an overnight hospital stay after each treatment is not a bad idea so that any side-effects can be dealt with quickly.

Side-effects of chemotherapy The most worrying effect of chemotherapy is possible damage to the bone marrow that replenishes blood cells; white cells are the most vulnerable. To check that levels of white blood cells remain normal and the body's immune system is intact, a blood sample will be taken before each treatment. If the white-cell count is too low, your next course of treatment will be put off or the dose reduced until the white-cell count returns to a safe level. Antibiotics or a blood transfusion during a course of chemotherapy may be needed to ameliorate this side-effect.

Other side-effects include tiredness, nausea, some hair loss, mouth ulcers, loss of appetite and diarrhoea. Any or all of these can make you feel miserable and ill. Simple remedies such as mouthwashes can help to combat mouth soreness, and powerful drugs have been specially developed to stop the nausea associated with the treatment. If your appetite is affected, whether it is suppressed or increased, your doctor or special-care nurse will be able to advise you about your diet. Some foods have been found to react with the drugs used in chemotherapy, but this is rare.

Given correctly, anti-cancer drugs need not necessarily cause complete hair loss, although you may find that your hair thins a little during the treatment. For some women, this is the most distressing side-effect, especially coming on top of the trauma of disfiguring breast surgery. Your hair will grow back after treatment or even before the treatment is completely finished, but it may be a little more curly and may have changed slightly in colour.

Anti-cancer drugs can often disrupt menstruation, and it may stop altogether. About 40 percent of women who are treated with chemotherapy will become infertile, and you should discuss this possibility with your doctor before treatment begins. The younger you are, the more likely your periods are to resume when chemotherapy ends.

STEM-CELL TREATMENT

About 17 years ago, it appeared that women with advanced breast cancer who received very high doses of chemotherapy were likely to live longer. However, doses of the cytotoxic drugs used are constrained by the poisonous effect on bone marrow.

- *To combat this, researchers developed a procedure that is called autologous stem-cell transfusion. This uses the woman's own bone marrow to rescue her from otherwise toxic high doses of chemotherapy.*

- *Stem cells, the cells that produce all other blood cells, are removed from the patient's blood or bone marrow and frozen. Then a course of high-dose chemotherapy is given over a period of four to five days in doses that would usually be sufficient to kill the stem cells (leading ultimately to the patient's death).*

- *Doctors can reinfuse the previously harvested stem cells after chemotherapy is complete. Because these cells have not been affected by chemotherapy, they can once again begin to form healthy blood cells.*

- *Stem-cell treatment remains controversial, traumatic and very expensive. It is not generally available in Europe, although it is in some centres in the US. In addition, the procedure is unfortunately not as successful as was first hoped.*

BREAST RECONSTRUCTION

If you have lost part or all of your breast, you can have reconstructive surgery. This involves the creation of a natural-looking artificial breast through plastic surgery. Although a reconstructed breast may look very real, there will be little or no feeling in the transferred skin. The psychological benefits and increased confidence you will experience in the way you look tend to outweigh the disadvantage of reduced sensation of the nipple and areola.

Every woman has the right to consult a specialist about reconstruction. If your doctor is reluctant to consider the option, seek a second opinion. Even the most well-adjusted woman flinches at the thought of mastectomy. It's reasonable to see the changes you have to make to the way you dress and to your lifestyle as a threat to your femininity and body-image. Above all the mastectomy scar may serve as a reminder of the cancer you once had. Reconstruction can go a long way to making you feel whole again. You'll no longer need prostheses (false breasts) or special bras, or feel so restricted in the kind of clothes you wear. Reconstruction can contribute a great deal to your self-esteem and your optimism about the future. About half of all mastectomy patients choose to have breast reconstruction, finding that it helps them to put their cancer behind them.

Reconstruction in no way restricts the treatments open to you. It doesn't interfere with radiotherapy, chemotherapy or hormone therapy. Post-operative follow-up is made no harder and recurrence can still be easily detected.

TIMING

Some consideration should be given to the timing of reconstruction. It may be possible for you to have it immediately after your mastectomy and under the same anaesthetic, or at any time afterwards. This means that a woman who had a mastectomy many years ago when breast reconstruction was not available can opt to have it now.

With immediate reconstruction you will wake from your operation with your breast still present even though it will have altered. The psychological stress associated with breast removal is greatly reduced and, in addition, you don't have to cope with the prospect of more surgery later.

Despite these advantages, immediate reconstruction isn't carried out very frequently because it involves two specialist surgeons (a cancer surgeon and a plastic surgeon) working together at the same time. This makes it a lengthy, difficult and complicated operation. There's also evidence that some women are less happy with the reconstructed breast if the reconstruction is done as part of the mastectomy operation, and some surgeons prefer waiting several months to make sure that the breast has healed completely.

You may not be able to take advantage of immediate reconstruction in the clinic that you attend but, if this is what you want, it may be possible for you to be transferred to a specialist breast unit that does offer it.

SUITABILITY FOR RECONSTRUCTION

Don't worry if you are slightly unfit; reconstructive surgery can be performed on any woman except the very frail. Even if you have widespread disease, your life expectancy may still be several years and the quality of your life during this time can be greatly improved by reconstruction.

Although half of all breast cancer patients will not need a mastectomy, even women who have conservative surgery may lose quite a lot of breast tissue. They too can take advantage of reconstructive surgery.

METHODS OF RECONSTRUCTION

Reconstructive surgery remoulds your breast mound, areola and nipple. The mound can be reconstructed using your own tissue (see p. 84) or an artificial implant. Two kinds of implant are available: fixed-volume implants and tissue expanders. Both types have a textured silicone shell filled with either saline (salt in solution) or silicone gel.

It's important to realize that the link between silicone implants and cancer is entirely unproven. Bear in mind, too, that implants have been around for more than 30 years and have been used in nearly two million women, not to mention the large number of people who use other silicone products, for instance contact lenses. In 1989, the FDA (Food and Drug Administration) in the US concluded that "a carcinogenic [cancer-producing] effect in humans could not be completely ruled out, but if such an effect did exist, the risk would be very low". Breast surgeons in the rest of the world have found this statement sufficiently reassuring to go on using silicone implants (continued p. 84).

ARTIFICIAL IMPLANTS

A fixed-volume implant is placed behind the muscles of the chest wall. Although this is the simplest operation, it's not suitable for all women since there may not be enough skin in the breast area to accommodate the implant.

If too little skin remains after your mastectomy to cover a fixed-volume implant, your doctor may recommend an expander implant (see right) – an empty sac with a hollow tube and small valve attached that is placed behind the muscles of the chest wall in the same way as a fixed-volume implant. Over a period of several months, your doctor will gradually fill the implant (through its attached valve) with saline solution, allowing the skin to stretch so that a fixed-volume implant may eventually be inserted.

YOUR OWN TISSUE

The simplest kind of breast reconstruction is carried out with an implant but there are several methods that use your own tissue. These reconstruction procedures (see right) all involve "flaps" and produce a better result than implants.

Skin, muscle and fat are taken as a flap from either your back or your abdomen. The flap from your back is called the latissimus dorsi flap; the flap from your abdomen is known as the rectus abdominis or TRAM (transverse rectus abdominis myocutaneous) flap. In this procedure, tissues with their arteries and veins intact are swivelled up to your breast area so that they can "take" in a similar way to a skin graft. The flap is tunnelled underneath your skin to the breast area and is fashioned into a breast mound resembling your other breast as closely as possible. Many women find implants of their own tissue preferable to the artificial kinds. However, these breast reconstructions require quite complex surgery, and occasionally there are side-effects such as a weakening of the abdominal muscles if a large amount of tissue has to be moved.

The final kind of reconstruction takes tissue from your buttocks as a free flap – the gluteus maximus flap. In this procedure, blood vessels supplying the tissue that is moved are cut and rejoined to blood vessels in the chest wall where the implant is placed. This is the most complex kind of reconstruction and for some patients it may be the most satisfactory. There is a small risk that the blood vessels will fail to join, in which case the implant may not take.

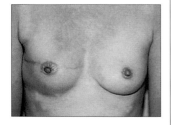

Reconstructed breast
In this example of a reconstruction, both the right breast and nipple have been reconstructed after a total mastectomy.

RECONSTRUCTION PROCEDURES

Tissue expander implant

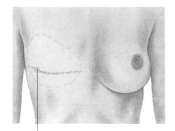

Valve under the skin allows saline to be injected later

Artificial implant
A hollow sac with a valve is put in place. Over a period of months, saline fluid is injected into the valve, allowing the skin to stretch gradually and naturally. The expander implant can then be replaced with a fixed-volume implant.

Latissimus dorsi flap (own tissue implant)

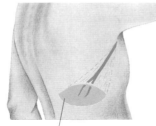

Section of skin, muscle and fat to be moved

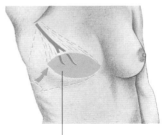

Flap brought under skin to front of chest

1 A flap of skin, muscle and fat is taken from the latissimus dorsi muscle on the back. The section of tissue to be moved keeps its feeding artery and blood vessels intact even after it has been moved to the new site.

2 The flap is tunnelled under the skin to the site of the mastectomy scar and the fat and muscle are fashioned into a mound. The new breast is stitched into place and the incision in the back is closed.

Rectus abdominis flap

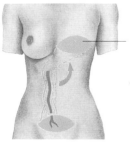

Flap is tunnelled into new position

Own tissue implant
A flap is taken from the rectus abdominis muscle, keeping its blood supply intact (the blood vessels are not cut). The flap is tunnelled under the skin to its new position. The incision in the abdomen is closed after the new breast mound has been stitched into place.

Gluteus maximus flap (own tissue implant)

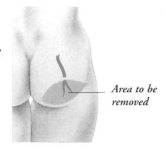

Area to be removed

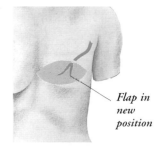

Flap in new position

1 A flap of skin, muscle and fat is removed from the gluteus maximus muscle in the buttocks. Its feeding artery is severed so that the flap can simply be placed in position without having to be tunnelled under the skin as for other procedures.

2 The flap is transferred to the mastectomy scar site and microsurgery is used to connect its blood vessels to those behind the muscles in the chest. The new breast mound is then stitched into place and the incision in the buttocks is closed.

THE IMPACT OF TREATMENT

A diagnosis of breast cancer and its treatment – especially if it involves the loss of a breast – still brings havoc in its wake. Despite the advent of surgical techniques that aim to conserve the breast, rates of anxiety and depression are still high. Women are just as anxious about having cancer as they are about the potential loss of a breast.

Nor are the psychological problems necessarily less if you have a lumpectomy rather than a mastectomy. For doctors to believe that your fears are minor compared with those of a woman facing a mastectomy could cause problems that may continue throughout your treatment, even into the follow-up period. Your feeling that you shouldn't bother your doctors with your fears may also reflect the popular expectation that women should be unreasonably stoical in the face of both physical and emotional pain.

A woman with breast cancer who's had a lumpectomy shouldn't have to handle the disease with cheerfulness and fortitude. Nor should just having a "little lump" removed create the feeling that, since treatment was comparatively trivial, you should quickly return to a normal psychological state; if you can't, you could end up feeling worthless and depressed. A pre-operative psychological test can identify 90 percent of women who'll become anxious and depressed in the year after surgery, enabling proper follow-up and help to be offered. If you feel vulnerable, ask for a test using the HAD (Hospital Anxiety and Depression) scale.

RADIOTHERAPY

Radiotherapy can involve daily treatment for up to six weeks. The greater the amount of radiation, the greater the chance of side-effects (see p. 79), which can be draining. If you are pre-menopausal, you may be worried that radiation will prevent you from having children; this isn't true. When doctors try to help with comments like "it's an insurance policy just to be sure we've got all the cancer", they can create doubts in your mind rather than reassuring you. Just the thought of having radiotherapy can sometimes be enough to produce side-effects. The more you understand the rationale behind your treatment and how it works, the less anxious you will be.

"My husband was just great, really supportive. I know that he was far more worried that I had a life-threatening disease than about the loss of my breast. But our sex life has changed, of course it has. I can't rid myself of the idea that really he hates my scar but is just trying to pretend that he doesn't mind."

Cheryl, 36, Musician

CHEMOTHERAPY

Chemotherapy has the worst reputation of all breast-cancer treatments because it's nearly always accompanied by some side-effects (see p. 81), including increased risk of infection.

For a woman who is feeling emotionally and physically bruised, the prospect of going through several courses of chemotherapy can cause a mixture of fear and suspicion. As with radiotherapy, the need for chemotherapy sometimes provokes fears that the cancer has not been totally removed.

Understandably you'll get more anxious and depressed if you have troublesome side-effects. It's a mistake to believe that a treatment must hurt to be effective, and it won't be stopped if you disclose your distress and discomfort to your doctors and care-givers. Tell them, and they will do all they can to give you the help and support you need.

SEXUAL RELATIONSHIPS

Powerful stereotyping in our society means that women's breasts have become symbolically linked to motherhood, femininity and sexuality. Don't feel inadequate if breast loss causes you severe sexual disturbance together with lowered self-esteem, loss of perceived attractiveness, embarrassment or inhibition and loss of sex drive. About one in five women has a loss of sexual interest a few months after mastectomy, and at two years the figure rises to one in three.

Interest in sex declines in over a quarter of sexually active women irrespective of the kind of surgical treatment they have. If you've had adjuvant therapy (see pp. 77–81), you're particularly vulnerable and likely to express more concern about physical affection, sexual relationships and lost feelings of femininity or sexual attractiveness.

Following radiotherapy, you may lose a lot of sensation in the affected breast. If your breasts were an important source of sexual stimulation prior to surgery, you'll need help and counselling to find another means of enhancing your enjoyment of lovemaking. Your partner may worry about being exposed to radiation by touching your breast while you are undergoing radiotherapy. This is not a danger.

The psychological impact of the diagnosis of cancer and treatment may make you so overwhelmingly preoccupied with thoughts of survival that sexual desire is at the bottom of your list of priorities. For some couples, however, the trauma of breast cancer can bring them closer together.

BODY IMAGE

Decisions about treatment are too often based on assumptions that older or sexually inactive women won't mind losing a breast. In one study of 62 women, more than half of those who chose lumpectomy were over the age of 50 and more than a quarter were over 60, demonstrating that age is not an acceptable criterion for deciding treatment.

• *You may become extremely self-conscious after mastectomy. Some women feel sure that people can tell they have only one breast, and become so distressed that they withdraw from the company of others. Up to one-third of post-mastectomy patients are unhappy with their prosthesis (see p. 89).*

• *Although mastectomy clearly has the greatest impact on how you perceive your body, not every woman who has breast conservation is pleased with the cosmetic outcome.*

• *Some women feel that being told they would have only the lump removed was misleading, since they expected to be left with symmetrical breasts. Unfortunately the necessary surgical procedure (called wide local excision) does not always fulfil these ideals.*

CHOOSING BRAS

Once your permanent prosthesis has been fitted, there's no reason why you shouldn't wear a wide variety of bras. The exceptions include styles that are wide on the shoulders and low cut, such as a half-cup bra. It's best to choose a cotton bra so that sweat can evaporate and your skin doesn't get hot and sticky under the prosthesis.

There are many attractive bras available with specially fitted pockets to hold your prosthesis in place, ensuring that it does not slip. Extra support in the rib-band and wide, supportive shoulder straps are important for comfort and can help your posture, which can be affected by a mastectomy.

LIFE AFTER TREATMENT

When treatment for breast cancer is complete, the story doesn't simply end. Rigorous follow-up will be necessary to pick up any problems and to check for any recurrence of the cancer. Having a mastectomy means that there are adjustments to make: you have to get used to a prosthesis and exercises to make your arm muscles strong. Then you have to learn to live with your new body. Even when treatment is complete, you could have psychological difficulties. After months of intensive medical attention you may feel alone and fearful, especially knowing there is no guarantee of a cure. This is a time when a care network such as a local breast-cancer group can be invaluable.

LYMPHOEDEMA

Disfigurement caused by surgery is not the only possible trauma you may face. Lymphoedema – painful swelling of the arm caused by radical radiotherapy or surgery on the axilla – can occasionally arise after treatment.

Healthy lymph nodes act as filters for the body's lymph fluid (see p. 10). Surgery can cause scarring of the nodes and this results in a blockage of the drainage system. The fluid stagnates in the arm, causing swelling and stiffness, which may be accompanied by a painful shoulder and possibly by nerve pain. With modern surgical techniques, lymphoedema is now rare and only five percent of mastectomy patients suffer from it to any degree. Severe lymphoedema hardly ever occurs.

Prevention and treatment   After the removal of your lymph nodes, you become more susceptible to infection, so you should protect your arm from knocks and scrapes, and wear gloves for rough household chores, gardening or any other work where your skin could be chafed.

It's important for you to do your post-mastectomy exercises regularly (see p. 90), since this can help to reduce the swelling by encouraging lymph drainage. Whenever you can, keep your arm raised, even when you're in bed or sitting on a sofa. Put your arm on a pile of cushions to keep it at about the same level as your neck. This will reduce swelling in your arm and help to build on the good work started by your daily exercises. If you have problems overnight with tingling in the fingers, try wearing an elastic bandage to prevent your arm from swelling.

PROSTHESES

A prosthesis is a false breast without a nipple but with an axillary tail, which resembles the texture, fullness and shape of a natural breast. You can wear a lightweight, temporary one as soon as your scar is healed, and then can be fitted with a permanent one to fit comfortably into your bra.

Every woman has the right to a good prosthesis. With the help of your surgeon, breast-care nurse or specially trained counsellor, you should easily be able to obtain one and even try various types to find the one that feels right.

If at first you can't find your ideal prosthesis, don't be disheartened. No prosthesis can fully replace your breast, but there's a good one for every woman who has had a mastectomy. Many kinds let you wear a swimsuit and low necklines without anyone being any the wiser, and you'll soon feel quite confident with your new shape. (There's a range of quite discreet prostheses for women whose breasts are asymmetrical following conservative surgery.)

BREAST PROSTHESES

A permanent prosthesis is made from silicone. It "gives" to the touch and feels heavy, just like a natural breast. A lightweight foam prosthesis has a hollow back that allows air to circulate. It can be useful as a temporary measure, for night wear and sports, or for very hot days when a permanent prosthesis can feel sticky and uncomfortable.

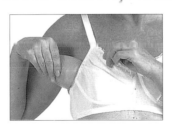

Fitting a prosthesis
Slip the prosthesis into the special pocket inside your bra. Make sure that it fills the cup and your underarm area.

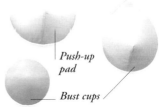

Push-up pad

Bust cups

Bra fillers
A variety of push-up pads and bust cups is available to fill out your bra after partial mastectomy.

Silicone prosthesis
Soft to the touch, a silicone prosthesis has the weight and droop of a natural breast.

Silicone nipples adhere to the prosthesis when moistened

TINTED PROSTHESIS	TRIANGULAR FORM	UNDERARM EXTENSION	TEARDROP SHAPE	LIGHTWEIGHT FORM

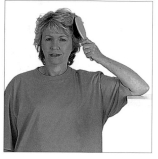

Hair brushing
Rest your arm on a firm surface. Keeping your head and shoulders upright, brush your hair upwards and sideways.

Arm circling
Stand as here, or sideways on to a firm table, leaning on it with your good arm. Bending slightly at the waist, let your affected arm hang loosely. Swing it forwards, backwards, left and right, and then in small circles.

POST-MASTECTOMY EXERCISES

You may find that your shoulder movement is restricted immediately following your operation. Normal movement and flexibility should gradually return, however, with the help of a few simple exercises, which are shown here.

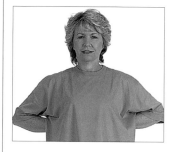

Bra fastening
Bend your arms at the elbows, keeping them at right angles to your body. Reach behind your back at bra level while slowly bringing your hands in towards your body. Relax from this position and begin again.

Towelling
Hold a towel or scarf stretched diagonally behind your back. Move it up and down along the line of the diagonal as if you were drying your back. Repeat with the towel or scarf held the other way.

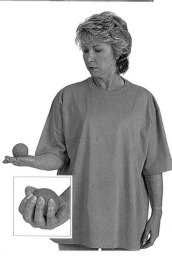

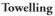

Lay your good arm on a flat surface

Hand squeezing
Hold a rubber ball on your flat palm. It should be firm enough so you have to exert pressure to squeeze it, but "give" enough for you to notice any improvement in muscle strength. Forming a fist around the ball, gently squeeze, then release. Repeat, but stop if you begin to ache.

As your arm relaxes, slowly increase the size of the swings

RECURRENCE AND RISK

Your age, menopausal status, the stage of the disease and the status of your axillary nodes will all have a profound affect on your initial chances of survival. In very general terms, women developing breast cancer under the age of 35 do less well than those whose breast cancer starts around the time of the menopause. Women between the ages of 35 and 50 who have not yet started the menopause do best. This means that many, many women have a good chance of surviving breast cancer, especially if it is detected early.

After successful treatment for breast cancer you will be concerned about how carefully you'll be followed up and how long it will be before you can be considered cured. The longer you live without a recurrence, the longer you will remain cancer-free, and the higher the chances of a cure. Because of this, most doctors believe that you should be carefully monitored for at least five years after treatment to detect possible recurrences or secondary spread.

You must be followed up for longer than five years before you can be said to be cured. Survival beyond ten years without any evidence of recurrence or spread would lead a doctor to be optimistic that you were cured, although women who have had breast cancer may still have a very small increased chance of dying from it, even 40 years after treatment, compared with healthy women of the same age.

TYPES OF RECURRENCE

There are three ways in which cancer can recur in the breast area. The most common recurrence is in the conserved breast in the region of the original cancer. This is not necessarily too serious; it's seen as cancer that is left over from the original treatment rather than as a secondary tumour. Since the cancer has not spread around the body, this type of recurrence is usually treated with a mastectomy.

Another kind of local recurrence concerns the lymph nodes (it affects only two percent of women). In general, it is not considered to be a sign of the cancer having spread and is therefore treated with further surgery or radiotherapy.

A recurrence of cancer in the scar or chest wall following a mastectomy is more serious. Because all your breast tissue has been removed, it is impossible for the cancer to be residual, and it must therefore have travelled from the lymphatic system or the bloodstream. Such recurrence, or

TREATMENT FOR RECURRENCE

Cancer can recur in the area of the treated breast regardless of the initial treatment. This happens in two or three cases out of ten, but is not a reason to be terrified or despondent.

Radiotherapy can cure any local recurrence, which is why follow-up schedules for patients must be strictly adhered to. A recurrence can then be detected so early that a relatively small dose of radiotherapy is all that is needed to eradicate it.

Bear in mind that mastectomy has a slightly lower risk of local recurrence than lumpectomy: mastectomy has a recurrence rate of 5–15 percent, whereas with lumpectomy the rate is 10–30 percent. In addition, radiotherapy following a lumpectomy is frequently given at the total body dose. This may mean that radiotherapy is no longer an option for treating a recurrence of breast cancer.

recurrence in your other breast or elsewhere in your body, is considered a secondary tumour, and will certainly require rigorous attention to curb the spreading cancer.

PREVIOUS BREAST CANCER AND RISK

A woman who has already had cancer of one breast is at a higher than average risk of developing cancer of the other breast, and this is why women who have had breast cancer must be meticulous about doing BSE on their remaining breast. Tamoxifen (see p. 79) seems to reduce the risk of a secondary cancer developing regardless of whether adjuvant treatment has been given, and in women with several risk factors tamoxifen might be considered as a preventive treatment. You should discuss this with your doctor.

As well as doing BSE (see pp. 16–17), you should also have regular mammograms performed on your remaining breast, because about 7 out of 100 women may develop a second primary tumour at some time in the future. A reasonable schedule for follow-up mammography would be six-monthly for two years and every 12 months thereafter.

THE REMAINING BREAST

Doctors can't agree whether the opposite breast should be biopsied at the time of initial surgery or during follow-up. Performing these biopsies might detect a good number of in situ lesions (see p. 54) that, if left alone, would cause no problems at all. On the other hand, since only a very small sample of breast tissue is taken during a biopsy, it's possible to miss some invasive cancers that are present.

An interesting study has been done on women under 65 with Stage I or II breast cancers (see p. 60) – that is, early cancer. When the opposite breast was biopsied, nearly one in six women were found to have some cancerous changes at the time of finding the first tumour. The vast majority of them, however, proved to be cancers that might never have become symptomatic and certainly would not kill. So these findings are of doubtful significance and it's still not clear which patients need treatment for them.

Such obsessive searching for cancers can lead to intense and unnecessary anxiety, and a wise course to pursue seems to be to monitor the remaining breast during follow-up sessions and reserve biopsy for any suspicious physical or mammographic findings. Do not hesitate to discuss with your doctor any uncertainties or worries you may have.

GLOSSARY

This list includes unfamiliar words and abbreviations that occur in this book, or that you may hear used by doctors and medical staff. Many of the terms are explained in more detail in the relevant chapters.

Ablation Destruction by means of X-rays or laser beam.

Adjuvant Additional to, for example, as in adjuvant therapy (see pp. 77–81).

Axilla The armpit.

Bilateral Both sides, as in affecting both breasts.

Biopsy Taking a specimen of tissue to make a precise diagnosis (as in a cutting-needle biopsy, see p. 58).

BSE Breast self-examination: regular checking of your breasts by looking and feeling (see pp. 16–17).

Calcification Deposits of calcium in a breast lump that show up on a mammogram as white dots (see also **microcalcifications**).

Carcinoma Cancer.

Contracture Hardening of scar tissue around a breast implant.

Cyst A benign, fluid-filled lump.

Cytology Examining cells from a lump or cyst for any evidence of cancer, as in **FNAC** (fine-needle aspiration cytology).

Ectasia Dilatation of the milk ducts behind the nipple.

Fibroadenoma A harmless lump formed during the natural growth cycle of a breast lobule.

Fistula An abnormal opening, such as from a chronic abscess to the skin or into a milk duct (as in nipple fistula).

FNAC Fine-needle aspiration cytology: a technique for sampling the cells in a breast lump (see p. 33).

Granuloma A small lump resulting from a chronic inflammation.

Histology The study of tissues under a microscope. The tissue comes from a **biopsy** specimen.

Hormone A chemical messenger from one part of the body that circulates in the bloodstream and exerts an effect on another part of the body.

Hyperplasia Excessive cell growth (see p. 53).

Impalpable Cannot be felt.

In situ cancer Non-invasive cancer confined to the area in which it arises. It does not spread and is not fatal.

Involution Dying back, shrinking, as in **ectasia** (see also p. 36).

Lesion Any newly-formed abnormal structure in the body.

Lobule The glandular part of the breast where milk is produced.

Luteal phase The second half of the menstrual cycle after ovulation has occurred.

Lymph nodes or glands The junctions of the lymphatic system (see p. 10) that become enlarged if fighting an infection or cancer.

Lymphoedema Swelling, pain and stiffness of the arm and hand, as a result of interference with the lymphatic drainage (see also p. 10) of the **axilla** following surgery and, more frequently, radiotherapy. This condition is now quite rare.

Mastitis Inflammation of breast tissue caused by infection.

Metastasis Spread of cancer to a distant part of the body where it forms a secondary tumour.

Microcalcifications Minute calcium deposits that have a white speckled appearance on mammography.

Micrometastasis A secondary tumour formed from only one or two cells that have escaped from the primary **tumour**.

Oncogene A cancer-promoting gene.

Oncology The study of cancer. An oncologist is a specialist in cancer and cancer treatments.

Peau d'orange Literally "orange peel". Dimpling of the skin caused by a breast **tumour** spreading upwards to tether the skin.

Pedicle A stalk.

Prosthesis An artificial or replacement body-part, as in breast prosthesis.

Quadrantectomy An operation that removes a quarter of the breast.

Radiologist A specialist who takes and interprets X-rays.

Radiotherapist A specialist who administers radiotherapy.

Tumour A new lump that can be benign or malignant.

Wide excision Cutting out a lump with a minimum of 1 centimetre (½ inch) of tissue around it.

USEFUL ADDRESSES

BREAST CARE

National Screening Co-ordination Office
Tel: 0114 282 0357

Women's Health
52 Featherstone Street
London EC1Y 8RT
Tel: 0845 1255254
Email: health@womenshealthlondon.org.uk
Website: www.womenshealthlondon.org.uk
Open Monday – Friday: 9.30 am – 1.30 pm
Counselling and literature; written health enquiry service

Women's Health Concern
P.O. Box 2126
Marlow
Buckinghamshire SL7 2RY
Tel: 01628 488065
Email: info@womens-health-concern.org
Website: www.womens-health-concern.org
Counselling and literature on all gynaecological problems, especially HRT (hormone replacement therapy)

CANCER

Against Breast Cancer
B363 Curie Avenue
Harwell International Business Centre
Oxfordshire OX11 0RA
Tel: 01235 820777
Email: info@aabc.org.uk
Website: www.aabc.org.uk

BACUP (British Association of
Cancer United Patients)
3 Bath Place, Rivington Street
London EC2A 3JR
Tel: 020 7696 9003
Helpline: 0808 800 1234
Email: see form on website (below)
Website: www.cancerbacup.org.uk

Breast Cancer Care
Kiln House
210 New Kings Road
London SW6 4NZ
Tel: 020 7384 2984
Helpline: 0808 800 6000
Email: info@breastcancercare.org.uk
Website: www.breastcancercare.org.uk
Counselling and literature

Bristol Cancer Help Centre
Grove House
Cornwallis Grove
Clifton
Bristol BS8 4PG
Tel: 0117 980 9500
Helpline: 0117 980 9500
Email: form on website (below)
Website: www.bristolcancerhelp.org
Complementary therapies for people with cancer

Cancer Research UK
P.O. Box 123
Lincoln's Inn Fields
London WC2A 3PX
Tel: 020 7242 0200
Email: form on website (below)
Website: www.cancerresearch.uk.org
Information, not advice

Macmillan CancerLine
Tel: 0808 808 2020
Website: www.cancerlink.org

Marie Curie Cancer Care
89 Albert Embankment
London SE1 7TP
Tel: 020 7599 7777
Email: info@mariecurie.org.uk
Website: www.mariecurie.org.uk
Education and practical nursing

COUNSELLING

British Association for Counselling (BAC)
1 Regent Place
Rugby
Warwickshire CV21 2PJ
Tel: 0870 443 5252
Email: bac@bac.org.uk
Website: www.counselling.co.uk

INDEX

ACKNOWLEDGMENTS

Dorling Kindersley would like to thank the following individuals and organizations for their contribution to this book.

PHOTOGRAPHY
All photographs by Debi Treloar and Ian Boddy except Mr. J. D. Frame, page 84; Eleanor Moskovic, The Royal Marsden NHS Trust, page 70; Science Photo Library/ Chris Priest, page 20

ILLUSTRATIONS AND CHARTS
Tony Graham, Paul Williams

MEDICAL CONSULTANT
Professor R. E. Mansel MS FRCS

ADVICE AND ASSISTANCE
Breast Cancer Care; Dr. Helena Earl, University Hospital Birmingham; Mr Ian Fentiman, Guy's Hospital; Mr. J. D. Frame FRCS, FRCS (Plast); Mr. Jerry Gilmore MS, FRCS, FRCS (Ed.); Professor Robert Mansel, University Hospital, Cardiff; Dr. Eleanor Moskovic MRCP, FRCR, The Royal Marsden NHS Trust; National Screening Co-ordination Office; Angela O'Grady, King's College Hospital; Patricia Paniale, Royal Free Hampstead NHS Trust; Professor R. D. Rubens MD, BSc, FRCP, Guy's Hospital; Professor

John Sloane, University of Liverpool; Mr. Meirion Thomas, The Royal Marsden NHS Trust; Dr. David Tong, Guy's Hospital

EQUIPMENT
The Bullen Health Care Group, Manchester; Nicola Jane, Chichester

ADDITIONAL EDITORIAL AND DESIGN ASSISTANCE
Nicky Adamson, Claire Cross, Ruth Tomkins

INDEX
Hilary Bird

TEXT FILM
The Brightside Partnership, London